T0250323

Biocomposites and Hybrid Biomaterials of Calcium Orthophosphates with Polymers

Biocomposites and Hybrid Biomaterials of Calcium Orthophosphates with Polymers

Sergey V. Dorozhkin

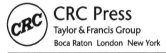

CRC Press
Taylor & Francis Group
Boca Raton London New York

CRC Press is an imprint of the
Taylor & Francis Group, an **Informa** business

CRC Press
Taylor & Francis Group
6000 Broken Sound Parkway NW, Suite 300
Boca Raton, FL 33487-2742

© 2019 by Taylor & Francis Group, LLC
CRC Press is an imprint of Taylor & Francis Group, an Informa business

No claim to original U.S. Government works

Printed on acid-free paper

International Standard Book Number-13: 978-1-138-34310-8 (Hardback)

Visit the Taylor & Francis Web site at
http://www.taylorandfrancis.com

and the CRC Press Web site at
http://www.crcpress.com

Contents

Preface

Various types of polymers have been widely used in long-term implants and controlled drug release applications. However, when it comes to tissue engineering, polymers suffer from some shortcomings such as slow degradation rates, poor mechanical properties, and low cell adhesion. The incorporation of calcium orthophosphates ($CaPO_4$) into polymers has yielded a number of biocomposites and hybrid biomaterials with remarkably improved mechanical properties, controllable degradation rates, as well as enhanced bioactivity and bioresorbability; all of these appear to be very important for bone tissue engineering. This book presents the state-of-the-art and recent advances in the fabrication and properties on biocomposites and hybrid biomaterials of $CaPO_4$ with polymers suitable for biomedical applications. Through the successful combinations of the desired properties of matrix materials with those of fillers (in such systems, both $CaPO_4$ and polymers may play either role), innovative bone graft biomaterials can be designed. Various types of $CaPO_4$/polymer formulations that are either already in use or being investigated for biomedical applications are discussed. The specific advantages of such formulations in the selected applications are highlighted. As the way from a laboratory to a hospital is a long one and the prospective biomedical candidates have to meet many different necessities, this book also examines the critical issues and scientific challenges that require further research and development.

Author

Sergey V. Dorozhkin received his MSc in chemical engineering with honors in 1984 from the Moscow Institute of Chemical Technology, Moscow, Russia, and his PhD in chemistry in 1992 from the Research Institute of Fertilizers, Moscow, Russia. From 1992 to 1994, he worked as a senior researcher at the same institute, and from 1994 to 1996, he worked as a biotechnologist at a Swiss–Russia joint venture. From 1996 to 2004, he held five postdoctoral positions in France, Portugal, Germany, and Canada, where he worked on various aspects of calcium orthophosphates. He has authored more than 70 research articles, approximately 30 reviews, 20 book chapters, and 4 monographs.

CHAPTER 1

Biocomposites and Hybrid Biomaterials of Calcium Orthophosphates (CaPO$_4$) with Polymers

1.1 INTRODUCTION

The fracture of bones due to various traumas or natural aging is a typical type of a tissue failure. An operative treatment frequently requires implantation of a temporary or a permanent prosthesis, which is still a challenge for orthopedic surgeons, especially in the cases of large bone defects. A fast aging of the population and serious drawbacks of natural bone grafts make the situation even worse; therefore, there is a high clinical demand for bone substitutes. Unfortunately, a medical application of xenografts (*e.g.*, bovine bone) is generally associated with potential viral infections.

In addition, xenografts have a low osteogenicity, an increased immunogenicity and, usually, resorb more rapidly than autogenous bone. Similar limitations are also valid for human allografts (*i.e.*, tissue transplantation between individuals of the same species but of nonidentical genetic composition), where the concerns about potential risks of transmitting tumor cells, a variety of bacterial and viral infections as well as immunological and blood group incompatibility are even stronger. Moreover, harvesting and conservation of allografts (exogenous bones) are additional limiting factors [1–3]. Autografts (endogenous bones) are still the "golden standard" among any substitution materials because they are osteogenic, osteoinductive, osteoconductive, completely biocompatible and nontoxic and do not cause any immunological problems (nonallergic). They contain viable osteogenic cells and bone matrix proteins and support bone growth. Usually, autografts are well accepted by the body and rapidly integrated into the surrounding bone tissues. Due to these reasons, they are used routinely for a long period with good clinical results [2–5]; however, it is fair to say on complication cases that frequently occurred in the past [6]. Unfortunately, a limited number of donor sites restrict the quantity of autografts harvested from the iliac crest or other locations of the patient's own body. In addition, their medical application is always associated with additional traumas and scars resulting from the extraction of a donor tissue during a superfluous surgical operation, which requires further healing at the donation site and can involve long-term postoperative pain. Thus, any types of biologically derived transplants appear to be imperfect solutions, mainly due to a restricted quantity of donor tissues, donor site morbidity as well as potential risks of an immunological incompatibility and disease transfer [7–9]. In this light, man-made materials (alloplastic or synthetic bone grafts) stand out as a reasonable option because they are easily available and might be processed and modified to suit the specific needs of a given application. What's more, there are no concerns about potential infections, immunological incompatibility, sterility and donor site morbidity. Therefore, investigations on artificial materials for bone tissue repair appear to be one of the key subjects in the field of biomaterials research for clinical applications [10,11].

Currently, there are several classes of synthetic bone grafting biomaterials for *in vivo* applications. The examples include natural coral, coral-derived materials, bovine porous demineralized bone, human demineralized bone matrix, bioactive glasses, glass–ceramics and $CaPO_4$ [12,13]. Among them, porous bioceramics made of $CaPO_4$ appear to be very prominent due to both the excellent biocompatibility and bonding ability to living bone in the body. This is directly related to the fact that the inorganic material of mammalian calcified tissues, that is, of bone and teeth, consists of $CaPO_4$ [14,15]. Due to this reason, other artificial materials are normally encapsulated by fibrous tissue, when implanted in body defects, while $CaPO_4$ are not. Many types of $CaPO_4$-based bioceramics with different chemical compositions are already on the market [16,17]. Unfortunately, as for any ceramic material, $CaPO_4$ bioceramics alone lack the mechanical and elastic properties of the calcified tissues. Namely, scaffolds made of $CaPO_4$ only suffer from a low elasticity, a high brittleness, a poor tensile strength, a low mechanical reliability and fracture toughness, which leads to various concerns about their mechanical performance after implantation. Besides, in many cases, it is difficult to form $CaPO_4$ bioceramics into the desired shapes [16,17].

The superior strength and partial elasticity of biological calcified tissues (*e.g.*, bones) are due to the presence of bioorganic polymers (mainly, collagen type I fibers) rather than due to a natural ceramic (mainly, a poorly crystalline ion-substituted calcium-deficient hydroxyapatite (CDHA), often referred to as "biological apatite") phase [18–21]. The elastic collagen fibers are aligned in bone along the main stress directions. The biochemical composition of bones is given in Table 1.1 [22]. A decalcified bone becomes very flexible and easily twisted, whereas a bone without collagen is very brittle; thus, the inorganic nano-sized crystals of biological apatite provide with the hardness and stiffness, while

TABLE 1.1 The Biochemical Composition[a] of Bones [22]

Inorganic Phases	wt%	Bioorganic Phases	wt%
$CaPO_4$ (biological apatite)	~60	Collagen type I	~20
Water	~9	Noncollagenous proteins: osteocalcin, osteonectin, osteopontin, thrombospondin, morphogenetic proteins, sialoprotein, serum proteins	~3
Carbonates	~4	Other traces: polysaccharides, lipids, cytokines	Balance
Citrates	~0.9	Primary bone cells: osteoblasts, osteocytes, osteoclasts	Balance
Sodium	~0.7		
Magnesium	~0.5		
Other traces: Cl^-, F^-, K^+ Sr^{2+}, Pb^{2+}, Zn^{2+}, Cu^{2+}, Fe^{2+}	Balance		

[a] The composition is varied from species to species and from bone to bone.

the bioorganic fibers are responsible for the elasticity and toughness. In bones, both types of materials integrate each other into a nanometric scale in such a way that the crystallite size, fiber orientation, short-range order between the components and so on determine its nanostructure and, therefore, the function and mechanical properties of the entire composite. From the mechanical point of view, bone is a tough material at low strain rates, but fractures more like a brittle material at high strain rates; generally, it is rather weak in tension and shear, particularly along the longitudinal plane. Besides, bone is an anisotropic material because its properties are directionally dependent [18–21].

It remains a great challenge to design the ideal bone graft that emulates nature's own structures or functions. Certainly, the successful design requires an appreciation of the bones' structure. According to expectations, the ideal bone graft should be benign; available in a variety of forms and sizes, all with sufficient mechanical properties for use in load-bearing sites; form a chemical bond at the bone/implant interface; as well as be osteogenic, osteoinductive, osteoconductive, biocompatible, completely bio-degradable at the expense of bone growth and moldable to fill and restore bone defects [23,24]. Furthermore, it should resemble the chemical composition of bones (thus, the presence of CaPO$_4$ is mandatory), exhibit contiguous porosity to encourage invasion by the live host tissue as well as possess both viscoelastic and semi-brittle behavior, as bones do [25–27]. Moreover, the degradation kinetics of the ideal implant should be adjusted to the healing rate of the human tissue with the absence of any chemical or biological irritation and/or toxicity caused by substances, which are released due to corrosion or degradation. Ideally, the combined mechanical strength of the implant and the ingrowing bone should remain constant throughout the regenerative process. Furthermore, the substitution implant material should not disturb significantly the stress environment of the surrounding living tissue [28]. Finally, there is an opinion that in the case of a serious trauma, bone should fracture rather than the implant [23]. A good sterilizability, stor-ability and processability as well as a relatively low cost are also of a great importance to permit a clinical application. Unfortunately, no artificial biomaterial is yet available, which embodies all these requirements, and unlikely, it will appear in the nearest future. To date, most of the available biomaterials appear to be either pre-dominantly osteogenic or osteoinductive or else purely osteocon-ductive [1].

Careful consideration of the bone type and mechanical properties is needed to design bone substitutes. Indeed, in high-load-bearing bones such as the femur, the stiffness of the implant needs to be adequate, not too stiff to result in strain shielding but rigid enough to present stability. However, in relatively low-load-bearing applications such as cranial bone repairs, it is more important to have stability and the correct three-dimensional (3D) shapes for aesthetic reasons. One of the most promising alternatives is to apply materials with similar composition and nanostructure to that of bone tissue. Mimicking the structure of calcified tissues and addressing the limitations of the individual materials, development of organic–inorganic hybrid biomaterials provides excellent possibilities for improving the conventional bone implants. In this sense, suitable biocomposites of tailored physical, biological and mechanical properties with the predictable degradation behavior can be prepared combining biologically relevant $CaPO_4$ with bioresorbable polymers [29]. As a rule, the general behavior of such biocomposites is dependent on nature, structure and relative contents of the constitutive components, although other parameters such as the preparation conditions also determine the properties of the final materials. Currently, $CaPO_4$ are incorporated as either a filler or a coating (or both) either into or onto a biodegradable polymer matrix, in the form of particles or fibers, and are increasingly considered for using as bone tissue engineering scaffolds due to their improved physical, biologic and mechanical properties [30–33]. In addition, such biocomposites could fulfill general requirements to the next generation of biomaterials that should combine the bioactive and bioresorbable properties to activate *in vivo* mechanisms of tissue regeneration, stimulating the body to heal itself and leading to replacement of the implants by the regenerating tissue. Thus, through the successful combinations of ductile polymer matrixes with hard and bioactive particulate bioceramic fillers, optimal materials can be designed, and ideally, this approach could lead to a superior construction to be used as either implants or posterior dental restorative material [29,34].

A lint-reinforced plaster was the first composite used in clinical orthopedics as an external immobilizer (bandage) in the treatment of bone fracture by Mathijsen in 1852 [35], followed by Dreesman in 1892 [36]. A great progress in the clinical application of various types of composite materials has been achieved since then. Based on both the past experience and the newly gained knowledge, various composite materials with tailored mechanical and biological performances can be manufactured and used to meet various clinical requirements [37]. However, this book presents only a brief history and advances in the field of $CaPO_4$-based biocomposites and hybrid biomaterials suitable for biomedical application. The majority of the reviewed literature is restricted to the recent publications; a limited number of articles published in the 20th century have been cited. Various aspects of the material constituents, fabrication technologies, structural and bioactive properties as well as phase interaction have been considered and discussed in detail. Finally, several critical issues and scientific challenges that are needed for further advancement are outlined.

1.2 GENERAL INFORMATION AND KNOWLEDGE

According to Wikipedia, the free encyclopedia, "*composite materials* (or *composites* for short) are engineered materials made from two or more constituent materials with significantly different physical or chemical properties and which remain separate and distinct on a macroscopic level within the finished structure" [38]. Thus, composites are always heterogeneous. Furthermore, the phases of any composite retain their identities and properties and are bonded, which is why an interface is maintained between them. This provides improved specific or synergistic characteristics that are not obtainable by any of the original phases alone [39]. Following the point of view of some predecessors, we also consider that "for the purpose of this review, composites are defined as those having a distinct phase distributed through their bulk, as opposed to modular or coated components" [40, page 1329]. For this reason, with a few important exceptions, the structures obtained by soaking of various materials in supersaturated solutions containing ions of calcium and orthophosphate (*e.g.*, Refs. [41–44]), those obtained by coating of various materials by CaPO$_4$ (reviewed in Refs. [45–47]) as well as CaPO$_4$ coated by other compounds [48–51] have not been considered; however, composite coatings have been considered. Occasionally, porous CaPO$_4$ scaffolds filled by cells inside the pores [52–55] as well as CaPO$_4$ impregnated by biologically active substances [56,57] are also defined as composites and/or hybrids; nevertheless, such structures have not been considered either.

In any composite, there are two major categories of constituent materials: a matrix phase (or a continuous phase) and a dispersed phase. To create a composite, at least one portion of each type is required. General information on the major fabrication and processing techniques might be found elsewhere [40,58]. The continuous phase is responsible for filling the volume, as well as it surrounds and supports the dispersed material(s) by maintaining their relative positions. The dispersed phase(s) is (are) usually responsible for enhancing one or more properties of the matrix. Most of the composites target an enhancement of mechanical properties of the matrix, such as stiffness and strength; however, other properties, such as erosion stability, transport properties (electrical or thermal), radiopacity, density or biocompatibility might also be of a great interest. This synergism produces the properties, which are unavailable from the individual constituent materials [58,59]. What's more, by controlling the volume fractions and local and global arrangements of the dispersed phase, the properties and design of composites can be varied and tailored to suit the necessary conditions. For example, in the case of ceramics, the dispersed phase serves to impede crack growth. In this case, it acts as reinforcement. A number of methods, including deflecting crack tips, forming bridges across crack faces, absorbing energy during pullout and causing a redistribution of stresses in regions, adjacent to crack tips, can be used to accomplish this [60]. Other factors to be considered in composites are the volume percentage of the dispersed phase(s), its(their) dimensions, shape and orientation, a reinforcement/matrix interfacial state as well as a homogeneity of the overall composite. For example, higher volume fractions of reinforcement phases tend to improve the mechanical properties of the composites, while continuous and aligned fibers best prevent crack propagation with the added property of anisotropic behavior. From a structural point of view, composites are anisotropic in nature: their mechanical properties are different in different directions. Furthermore, the uniform distribution of the dispersed phase is also desirable, as it imparts consistent properties to the composite [38,58,59].

In general, composites might be simple, complex, graded and hierarchical. The term "a simple composite" is referred to the composites that result from the homogeneous dispersion of one dispersed phase throughout a matrix. The term "a complex composite" is referred to the composites that result from the homogeneous dispersion of several dispersed phases throughout a matrix. The term "a graded composite" is referred to the composites that result from the intentionally structurally inhomogeneous dispersion of one or several dispersed phases throughout a matrix. The term "a hierarchical composite" is referred to the cases when fine entities of either a simple or a complex composite are somehow aggregated to form coarser ones (*e.g.*, granules or particles) which later are dispersed inside another matrix to produce the second hierarchical scale of the composite structure. There is another set of four types of composites: (i) fibrous composites, where the fibers are in a matrix; (ii) laminar composites, in which the phases are in layers; (iii) particulate composites, where the particles or flakes are in a matrix; and (iv) hybrid composites, which are combinations of any of the above. Still, other classification type of the available composites is based on the matrix materials (metals, ceramics and polymers) [37].

In most cases, three interdependent factors must be considered in designing of any composite: (i) a selection of the suitable matrix and dispersed materials; (ii) a choice of appropriate fabrication and processing methods; and (iii) both internal and external designs of the device itself [40]. Furthermore, any composite must be formed to shape. To do this, the matrix material can be added before or after the dispersed material has been placed into a mold cavity or onto the mold surface. The matrix material experiences a melding event, which, depending on the nature of the matrix material, can occur in various ways such as chemical polymerization, setting, curing or solidification from a melted state. Due to a general inhomogeneity, the physical properties of many composite materials are not isotropic but rather orthotropic (*i.e.*, there are different properties or strengths in different orthogonal directions) [38,58,59].

In order to prepare any type of a composite, at least two different materials must be mixed. Thus, a phase miscibility phenomenon appears to be of the paramount importance [61,62]. Furthermore, the interfacial strength among the phases is a very important factor because a lack of adhesion among the phases will result in an early failure at the interface and thus in a decrease in the mechanical properties, especially the tensile strength. From a chemical point of view, one can distinguish several types of the interactions among the composite components: materials with strong (covalent, coordination and ionic) interactions, with weak interactions (van der Waals forces, hydrogen bonds and hydrophilic–hydrophobic balance) or without chemical interactions among the components [63]. Wetting is also important in bonding or adherence of the materials. It depends on the hydrophilicity or polarity of the filler(s) and the available polar groups of the matrix.

Biocomposites are defined as nontoxic composites able to interact well with the human body *in vivo* and, ideally, contain one or more component(s) that stimulate(s) the healing process and uptake of the implant [64]. Thus, for biocomposites, the biological compatibility appears to be more important than any other type of compatibility [37,65–67]. Interestingly that according to the databases, the first article with the term "biocomposite" in the title was published in 1987 [68] and the one containing a combination of terms "biocomposite" and hydroxyapatite (HA) in the title was published in 1991 [69]. Thus, the subject of $CaPO_4$-based biocomposites and hybrid biomaterials appears to be quite new. The most common properties from the bioorganic and inorganic domains to be combined in biocomposites have been summarized in Table 1.2 [24]. For general advantages of the modern $CaPO_4$-based biocomposites over $CaPO_4$ bioceramics and bioresorbable polymers individually, the interested readers are advised to go through the "Composite materials strategy" section of Ref. [29].

TABLE 1.2   General Respective Properties from the Bioorganic and Inorganic Domains, to be Combined in Various Composites and Hybrid Materials [24]

Inorganic	Bioorganic
Hardness, brittleness	Elasticity, plasticity
High density	Low density
Thermal stability	Permeability
Hydrophilicity	Hydrophobicity
High refractive index	Selective complexation
Mixed valence slate (red-ox)	Chemical reactivity
Strength	Bioactivity

1.3 THE MAJOR CONSTITUENTS OF BIOCOMPOSITES AND HYBRID BIOMATERIALS FOR BONE GRAFTING

1.3.1 CaPO$_4$

CaPO$_4$ were first mentioned in 1769 as the major constituents of bones and have been investigated since then [70,71]. The main driving force behind the use of CaPO$_4$ as bone-substitute materials is their chemical similarity to the mineral component of mammalian bones and teeth [14–16]. As a result, in addition to being nontoxic, they are biocompatible, not recognized as foreign materials in the body, and most importantly, both exhibit bioactive behavior and integrate into living tissue by the same processes active in remodeling healthy bone. This leads to an intimate physicochemical bond between the implants and bone, termed osteointegration. More to the point, CaPO$_4$ are also known to support osteoblast adhesion and proliferation. Even so, the major limitations to use CaPO$_4$ as load-bearing biomaterials are their mechanical properties; namely, they are brittle with poor fatigue resistance [23]. The poor mechanical behavior is even more evident for highly porous ceramics and scaffolds because porosity greater than 100 μm is considered as the requirement for proper vascularization and bone cell colonization [72,73]. That is why, in biomedical applications, CaPO$_4$ are used primarily as fillers and coatings [16].

The complete list of known $CaPO_4$, including their standard abbreviations and the major properties, is given in Table 1.3, while the detailed information on $CaPO_4$ might be found in special books and monographs [16,74–78].

1.3.2 Polymers

Polymers are a class of materials consisting of large molecules, often containing many thousands of small units, or monomers, joined together chemically to form one giant chain, thus creating very ductile materials. In this respect, polymers are comparable with major functional components of the biological environment: lipids, proteins and polysaccharides. They differ from each other in chemical composition, molecular weight, polydispersity, crystallinity, hydrophobicity, solubility and thermal transitions. Besides, their properties can be fine-tuned over a wide range by varying the type of polymer and chain length as well as by copolymerization or blending of two or more polymers [79,80]. Opposite to ceramics, polymers exhibit substantial viscoelastic properties and easily can be fabricated into complex structures, such as sponge-like sheets, gels or complex structures with intricate porous networks and channels [81]. Being X-ray transparent and nonmagnetic, polymeric materials are fully compatible with the modern diagnostic methods such as computed tomography and magnetic resonance imaging. Unfortunately, most of them are unable to meet the strict demands of the *in vivo* physiological environment. Namely, the main requirements to polymers suitable for biomedical applications are that they must be biocompatible, not eliciting an excessive or chronic inflammatory response on implantation and, for those that degrade, that they breakdown into nontoxic products only. Unfortunately, polymers, for the most part, lack rigidity, ductility and ultimate mechanical properties required in load-bearing applications. Thus, despite their good biocompatibility, many of the polymeric materials are mainly used for soft tissue replacements (such as skin, blood vessel, cartilage, ligament replacement, *etc.*). Moreover, the sterilization

TABLE 1.3   Existing CaPO$_4$ and Their Major Properties [16]

Ca/P Molar Ratio	Compound	Formula	Solubility at 25°C, $-\log(K_s)$	Solubility at 25°C, g/L	pH Stability Range in Aqueous Solutions at 25°C
0.5	Monocalcium phosphate monohydrate (MCPM)	$Ca(H_2PO_4)_2 \cdot H_2O$	1.14	~18	0.0–2.0
0.5	Monocalcium phosphate anhydrous (MCPA or MCP)	$Ca(H_2PO_4)_2$	1.14	~17	a
1.0	Dicalcium phosphate dihydrate (DCPD), mineral brushite	$CaHPO_4 \cdot 2H_2O$	6.59	~0.088	2.0–6.0
1.0	Dicalcium phosphate anhydrous (DCPA or DCP), mineral monetite	$CaHPO_4$	6.90	~0.048	a
1.33	Octacalcium phosphate (OCP)	$Ca_8(HPO_4)_2(PO_4)_4 \cdot 5H_2O$	96.6	~0.0081	5.5–7.0
1.5	α-Tricalcium phosphate (α-TCP)	$\alpha\text{-}Ca_3(PO_4)_2$	25.5	~0.0025	b
1.5	β-Tricalcium phosphate (β-TCP)	$\beta\text{-}Ca_3(PO_4)_2$	28.9	~0.0005	b

(Continued)

TABLE 1.3 (*Continued*)   Existing CaPO$_4$ and Their Major Properties [16]

Ca/P Molar Ratio	Compound	Formula	Solubility at 25°C, −log(K_s)	Solubility at 25°C, g/L	pH Stability Range in Aqueous Solutions at 25°C
1.2–2.2	Amorphous calcium phosphates (ACP)	Ca$_x$H$_y$(PO$_4$)$_z$·nH$_2$O, $n=3$–4.5; 15%–20% H$_2$O	c	c	~5–12[d]
1.5–1.67	Calcium-deficient hydroxyapatite (CDHA or Ca-def HA)[e]	Ca$_{10-x}$(HPO$_4$)$_x$(PO$_4$)$_{6-x}$(OH)$_{2-x}$ (0 < x < 1)	~85	~0.0094	6.5–9.5
1.67	Hydroxyapatite (HA, HAp or OHAp)	Ca$_{10}$(PO$_4$)$_6$(OH)$_2$	116.8	~0.0003	9.5–12
1.67	Fluorapatite (FA or FAp)	Ca$_{10}$(PO$_4$)$_6$F$_2$	120.0	~0.0002	7–12
1.67	Oxyapatite (OA, OAp or OXA)[f], mineral voelckerite	Ca$_{10}$(PO$_4$)$_6$O	~69	~0.087	b
2.0	Tetracalcium phosphate (TTCP or TetCP), mineral hilgenstockite	Ca$_4$(PO$_4$)$_2$O	38–44	~0.0007	b

a   Table at temperatures above 100°C.
b   These compounds cannot be precipitated from aqueous solutions.
c   Cannot be measured precisely. However, the following values were found: 25.7 ± 0.1 (pH = 7.40), 29.9 ± 0.1 (pH = 6.00), 32.7 ± 0.1 (pH = 5.28). The comparative extent of dissolution in acidic buffer is ACP ≫ α-TCP ≫ β-TCP > CDHA ≫ HA ≫ FA.
d   Always metastable.
e   Occasionally, it is called "precipitated HA (PHA)."
f   Existence of OA remains questionable.

processes (autoclave, ethylene oxide and ^{60}Co irradiation) may affect the polymer properties [82]. There is a variety of biocompatible polymers suitable for biomedical applications [83–85]. For example, polyacrylates, poly(acrylonitrile-*co*-vinylchloride) and polylysine have been investigated for cell encapsulation and immunoisolation [86,87]. Polyorthoesters and poly(ε-caprolactone) (PCL) have been investigated as drug delivery devices, the latter for long-term sustained release because of their slow degradation rates [88]. PCL is an aliphatic linear polyester, bioresorbable and biocompatible polymer, having appropriate resorption period and releases nontoxic by-products on degradation. Therefore, it is generally used in pharmaceutical products and wound dressings [89,90]. Polyurethane (PU) is in use in engineering of both hard and soft tissues, as well as in nanomedicine [91]. Polymers considered for orthopedic purposes include polyanhydrides, which have also been investigated as delivery devices (due to their rapid and well-defined surface erosion), for bone augmentation or replacement since they can be photopolymerized *in situ* [88,92,93]. To overcome their poor mechanical properties, they have been copolymerized with imides or formulated to be cross-linkable *in situ* [93]. Other polymers, such as polyphosphazenes, can have their properties (*e.g.*, degradation rate) easily modified by varying the nature of their side groups and have been shown to support osteoblast adhesion, which makes them candidate materials for skeletal tissue regeneration [93]. Poly(propylene-*co*-fumarate) (PPF) has emerged as a good bone replacement material, exhibiting good mechanical properties (comparable to trabecular bone), possessing the capability to cross-link *in vivo* through the C=C bond and being hydrolytically degradable. It has also been examined as a material for drug delivery devices [88,92–95]. Polycarbonates have been suggested as suitable materials to make scaffolds for bone replacement and have been modified with tyrosine-derived amino acids to render them biodegradable [88,96]. Polydioxanone has also been tested for biomedical applications [97]. Polymethyl methacrylate (PMMA) is widely used in orthopedics, as bone cement for implant fixation, as well as to repair certain fractures and bone defects, for example, osteoporotic vertebral bodies [98,99]. However, PMMA sets by a polymerization of toxic monomers, which also evolves significant amounts of heat that damages tissues. Moreover, it is neither degradable nor bioactive, does not bond chemically to bones and might generate particulate debris leading to an inflammatory foreign body response [92,100]. A number of other nondegradable polymers applied in orthopedic surgery include polyethylene (PE) in its different modifications, such as low-density PE, high-density PE (HDPE) and ultrahigh-molecular-weight PE (used as the articular surface of total hip replacement implants [101,102]); polyethylene terephthalate; and polypropylene (PP), which are applied to repair knee ligaments [103]. Polyactive™, a block copolymer of polyethylene glycol (PEG) and polybutylene terephthalate (PBT), was also considered for biomedical application [104–106]. Cellulose [107,108] and its esters [109,110] are also popular. Finally yet importantly, polyethylene oxide, polyhydroxybutyrate (PHB) and blends thereof have also been tested for biomedical applications [29].

Nonetheless, the most popular synthetic polymers used in medicine are the linear aliphatic poly(α-hydroxyesters) such as polylactic acid (PLA), polyglycolic acid (PGA) and a series of their copolymers with tunable properties (*e.g.*, a degree of crystallinity and a degradation rate, depending on their specific composition) – poly(lactic-*co*-glycolic) acid (PLGA; Table 1.4). These materials are fully biobased and biodegradable thermoplastic polyesters, which can be produced from different renewable resources such as starch, corn and sugarcane. Currently, they are the second-most consumed bioplastics in the world due to their use as both commodity and specialty applications. These polyesters have been extensively studied; they appear to be the only synthetic and biodegradable polymers with an extensive Food and Drug Administration (FDA) approval history [29,93,111,112]. They are biocompatible, mostly noninflammatory as well as

TABLE 1.4 Major Properties of Several FDA Approved Biodegradable Polymers [111]

Polymer	Thermal Properties (°C)	Tensile Modulus (GPa)	Degradation Time (Months)
Polyglycolic acid (PGA)	$t_g = 35{-}40$ $t_m = 225{-}230$	7.06	6–12 (strength loss within 3 weeks)
L-Polylactic acid (LPLA)	$t_g = 60{-}65$ $t_m = 173{-}178$	2.7	>24
D,L-Polylactic acid (DLPLA)	$t_g = 55{-}60$ Amorphous	1.9	12–16
85/15 D,L-Polylactic-co-glycolic acid (85/15 DLPLGA)	$t_g = 50{-}55$ Amorphous	2.0	5–6
75/25 D,L-Polylactic-co-glycolic acid (75/25 DLPLGA)	$t_g = 50{-}55$ Amorphous	2.0	4–5
65/35 D,L-Polylactic-co-glycolic acid (65/35 DLPLGA)	$t_g = 45{-}50$ Amorphous	2.0	3–4
50/50 D,L-Polylactic-co-glycolic acid (50/50 DLPLGA)	$t_g = 45{-}50$ Amorphous	2.0	1–2
Poly(ε-caprolactone) (PCL)	$t_g = (-60){-}(-65)$ $t_m = 58{-}63$	0.4	>24

t_g: glass transition temperature; t_m, melting point.

degrade *in vivo* through hydrolysis and possible enzymatic action into products that are removed from the body by regular metabolic pathways [88,93,113]. Besides, they might be used for drug delivery purposes [114]. Poly(α-hydroxyesters) have been investigated as scaffolds for replacement and regeneration of a variety of tissues, cell carriers, controlled delivery devices for drugs or proteins (*e.g.*, growth factors), membranes or films, screws, pins and plates for orthopedic applications [88,93,115,116]. In addition, the degradation rate of PLGA can be adjusted by varying the amounts of the two component monomers (Table 1.4), which in orthopedic applications can be exploited to create materials that degrade in concert with bone ingrowth [117]. Furthermore, PLGA is known to support osteoblast migration and proliferation [93,118], which is a necessity for bone tissue regeneration. Unfortunately, such polymers on their own, though they reduce the effect of stress shielding, are too weak to be used in load-bearing situations and are only recommended in certain clinical indications, such as ankle and elbow fractures [113]. In addition, they exhibit bulk degradation, leading to both a loss in mechanical properties and lowering of the local solution pH that accelerates further degradation in an autocatalytic manner. As the body is unable to cope with the vast amounts of implant degradation products, this might lead to an inflammatory foreign body response. Finally, poly(α-hydroxyesters) do not possess the bioactive and osteoconductive properties [93,119].

Several classifications of the biomedically relevant polymers are possible. For example, some authors distinguish between synthetic polymers such as PE, PMMA, PLA, PGA and PCL and polymers of biological origin, which comprise polysaccharides (starch, alginate, chitin/chitosan [120,121], gellan gum, cellulose, hyaluronic acid and its derivatives), proteins (soy, collagen, gelatin, fibrin and silk) and a variety of biofibers, such as lignocellulosic natural fibers [122,123]. Among them, natural polymers often possess highly organized structures. In addition, they may contain an extracellular substance, called ligand, which is necessary to bind with cell receptors. However, they always contain various impurities, which should be removed prior use. As synthetic polymers can be produced under the controlled conditions, they, in general, exhibit predictable and reproducible mechanical and physical properties such as tensile strength, elastic modulus and degradation rate. Control of impurities is a further advantage of synthetic polymers. Other authors differentiate between resorbable or biodegradable (*e.g.*, poly(α-hydroxyesters), polysaccharides and proteins) and nonresorbable (*e.g.*, PE, PP, PMMA and cellulose) polymers [123]. Furthermore, polymeric materials can be broadly classified as thermoplastics and thermosets. For example, HDPE and polyetheretherketone (PEEK) are the examples of thermoplastics, while polydimethylsiloxane and PMMA are the examples of thermosets [82]. The list of synthetic biodegradable polymers used for biomedical application as scaffold materials is available as Table 1 in Ref. [123], while further details on polymers suitable for biomedical applications are available in the literature [82,116,124–129] where the interested readers are referred. Good reviews on the synthesis of various biodegradable polymers [130], application of biodegradable shape-memory polymers in medicine [131], as well as experimental trends in polymer composites [132], are available elsewhere.

1.4 BIOCOMPOSITES AND HYBRID BIOMATERIALS BASED ON CaPO$_4$

1.4.1 Biocomposites with Polymers

Given their inherent biomimicry, CaPO$_4$/polymer biocomposites and hybrid biomaterials have been investigated extensively for bone regeneration. In such formulations, hard and stiff CaPO$_4$ bioceramics provide building blocks that are essential for both the mechanical strength and biomineralization, while flexible and soft polymeric components comprise those that have shown a good biocompatibility and are routinely used in surgical applications. Thus, the formation of CaPO$_4$/polymer biocomposites and hybrid biomaterials capitalizes the advantages of both material types and minimizes their shortcomings. In general, since polymers have a low modulus (2–7 GPa, as the maximum) as compared to that of bones (3–30 GPa), in order to mimic the latter, $CaPO_4$ bioceramics need to be loaded at a high weight % ratio. Besides, general knowledge on composite mechanics suggests that any high aspect ratio particles, such as whiskers or fibers, significantly improve the modulus at a lower loading. Thus, some attempts have been already performed to prepare biocomposites containing whisker-like [133–139] or needle-like [140–143] $CaPO_4$, as well as $CaPO_4$ fibers [144].

The history of implantable $CaPO_4$/polymer formulations started in 1981 (however, a more general topic "ceramic-plastic material as a bone substitute" is, at least, 18 years older [145]) from the pioneering study by Prof. William Bonfield et al. at Queen Mary College, University of London, performed on HA/PE blends [146,147]. That initial study introduced a bone-analogue concept, when proposed biocomposites comprised a polymer ductile matrix of PE and a ceramic stiff phase of HA, and was substantially extended and developed in further investigations by that research group [66,148–158]. More recent studies included investigations on the influence of surface topography of HA/PE composites on cell proliferation and attachment [159–162]. The material is composed of a particular combination of HA particles at a volume loading of ~40% uniformly dispensed in an HDPE matrix. The idea was to mimic bones using a polymeric matrix that can develop a considerable anisotropic character through adequate orientation techniques reinforced with a bone-like bioceramics that assures both a mechanical reinforcement and a bioactive character of the composite. Following FDA approval in 1994, in 1995, this material has become commercially available under the trade name HAPEX™ (Smith & Nephew Richards, Bartlett, TN), and to date, it has been implanted in over 300,000 patients with the successful results. It remains the only clinically successful bioactive composite, which was a major step in the implant field [163]. The major production stages of HAPEX include blending, compounding and centrifugal milling. A bulk material or device is then created from this powder by compression and injection molding [37]. Besides, HA/HDPE biocomposites might be prepared by a hot rolling technique that facilitated uniform dispersion and blending of the reinforcements in the matrix [164]. In addition, PP might be used instead of PE [165–168].

A mechanical interlock between both the phases of HAPEX is formed by shrinkage of HDPE onto the HA particles during cooling [66,67,169]. Both HA particle size and their distribution in the HDPE matrix were recognized as important parameters affecting the mechanical behavior of HAPEX. Namely, smaller HA particles were found to lead to stiffer composites due to general increasing of interfaces between the polymer and the ceramics; furthermore, rigidity of HAPEX was found to be proportional to HA volume fraction [153]. Furthermore, coupling agents, for example, 3-trimethoxysilylpropyl methacrylate for HA and acrylic acid for HDPE, might be used to improve bonding (by both chemical adhesion and mechanical coupling) between HA and HDPE [170,171]. Obviously, other types of CaPO$_4$ might be used instead of HA in biocomposites with PE [172]. Furthermore, attempts were performed to improve the mechanical properties of HAPEX by incorporating other ceramic phases into the polymer matrix, such as partially stabilized zirconia [173] and alumina [174]. For example, a partial replacement of HA filler particles by partially stabilized zirconia particles was found to lead to an increase in the strength and fracture toughness of HA/HDPE biocomposites. The compressive stress, set up by the volume expansion associated with tetragonal to monoclinic phase transformation of partially stabilized zirconia, inhibits or retards the crack propagation within the composite. This results in an enhanced fracture toughness of the HA/ZrO$_2$/HDPE biocomposite [173].

Various studies revealed that HAPEX attached directly to bones by chemical bonding (a bioactive fixation), rather than forming fibrous encapsulation (a morphological fixation). Initial clinical applications of HAPEX came in orbital reconstruction [175], but since 1995, the main uses of this composite have been in the shafts of middle ear implants for the treatment of conductive hearing loss [176,177]. In both applications, HAPEX offers the advantage of in situ shaping, so a surgeon can make final alterations to optimize the fit of the prosthesis to the bone of a patient, and subsequent activity requires only limited mechanical loading with virtually no risk of failure from insufficient tensile strength [66,67]. As compared to cortical bones, HA/PE composites have a superior fracture toughness for HA concentrations below ~40% and similar fracture toughness in the 45%–50% range. Their Young's modulus is in the range of 1–8 GPa, which is quite close to that of bone. The examination of the fracture surfaces revealed that only mechanical bond occurs between HA and PE. Unfortunately, the HA/PE composites are not biodegradable, the available surface area of HA is low and the presence of bioinert PE decreases the ability to bond to bones. Furthermore, HAPEX has been designed with a maximized density to increase its strength, but the resulting lack of porosity limits the ingrowth of osteoblasts when the implant is placed into the body [23]. Further details on HAPEX are available elsewhere [66,67]. Except HAPEX, other types of HA/PE biocomposites are also known [178–186].

Both linear and branched PEs were used as a matrix, and the biocomposites with the former were found to give a higher modulus [179]. The reinforcing mechanisms in $CaPO_4$/polymer formulations have yet to be convincingly disclosed. Generally, if a poor filler choice is made, the polymeric matrix might be affected by the filler through reduction of molecular weight during composite processing, formation of an immobilized shell of polymer around the particles (transcrystallization, surface-induced crystallization or epitaxial growth) and changes in conformation of the polymer due to particle surfaces and inter-particle spacing [66,67]. However, the reinforcing effect of $CaPO_4$ particles might depend on the molding technique employed: A higher orientation of the polymeric matrix was found to result in a higher mechanical performance of the composite [184,185].

Many other blends of CaPO$_4$ with various polymers are possible, including rather unusual formulations with dendrimers [187]. Even light-curable CaPO$_4$/polymer formulations are known [188]. The list of the appropriate CaPO$_4$ is shown in Table 1.3 (except monocalcium phosphate monohydrate (MCPM) and monocalcium phosphate anhydrous (MCPA) – both are too acidic and, therefore, are not biocompatible [16]; nevertheless, to overcome this drawback, they might be mixed with basic compounds, such as HA, tetracalcium phosphate (TTCP), CaCO$_3$, CaO, *etc.*); many biomedically suitable polymers have been listed above. The combination of CaPO$_4$ and polymers into biocomposites has a twofold purpose. The desirable mechanical properties of polymers compensate for a poor mechanical behavior of CaPO$_4$ bioceramics, while, in turn, the desirable bioactive properties of CaPO$_4$ improve those of polymers, expanding the possible uses of each material within the body [189–192]. Namely, polymers have been added to CaPO$_4$ in order to improve their mechanical strength [189], while CaPO$_4$ fillers have been blended with polymers to improve their compressive strength and modulus, in addition to increasing their osteoconductive properties [119,193–196]. In 1990s, it was established that with increasing of CaPO$_4$ content, both Young's modulus and bioactivity of the biocomposites generally increased, while the ductility decreased [23]. However, the later investigations revealed that the mechanical properties of CaPO$_4$/polymer biocomposites were not so straightforward: the strength was found to decrease with increasing the CaPO$_4$ content in such biocomposites [197]. Nevertheless, biocompatibility of such biocomposites is enhanced because CaPO$_4$ fillers induce an increased initial flash spread of serum proteins compared to the more hydrophobic polymer surfaces [198]. What's more, experimental results of these biocomposites indicated favorable cell–material interactions with increased cell activities as compared to each polymer alone [191]. Furthermore, such formulations can provide a sustained release of calcium and orthophosphate ions into the milieus, which is important for mineralized tissue regeneration [190]. Indeed, a combination of two different materials draws on the advantages of each one to create a superior biocomposite with respect to the materials on their own.

It is logical to assume that the proper biocomposite of a $CaPO_4$ (for instance, CDHA) with a bioorganic polymer (for instance, collagen) would yield the physical, chemical and mechanical properties similar to those of human bones. Different ways have been already realized to bring these two components together into biocomposites, such as mechanical blending, compounding, ball milling, dispersion of ceramic fillers into a polymer–solvent solution, a melt extrusion of a ceramic/polymer powder mixture, coprecipitation and electrochemical codeposition [22,37,199–201]. A total of three methods for preparing a homogeneous blend of HA with poly(L-lactic acid) (PLLA) were compared [199]. A dry process, consisting in mixing ceramic powder and polymer pellets before a compression-molding step, was used. The second technique was based on the dispersion of ceramic fillers into a polymer–solvent solution. The third method was a melt extrusion of a ceramic/polymer powder mixture. Mixing dry powders led to a ceramic particle network around the polymer pellets, whereas the solvent and melt methods also produced a homogeneous dispersion of HA in the matrix. The main drawback of the solvent casting method is the risk of potentially toxic organic solvent residues. The melt extrusion method was shown to be a good way to prepare homogeneous ceramic/polymer blends [199].

Besides, there is *in situ* formation, which involves either synthesizing the reinforcement inside a preformed matrix material or synthesizing the matrix material around the reinforcement [37,202,203]. This is one of the most attractive routes, since it avoids extensive particle agglomeration. For example, several articles have reported in situ formation technique to produce various composites of $CaPO_4$ with carbon nanotubes [204–207]. Other examples comprise using amino acid-capped gold nano-sized particles as scaffolds to grow CDHA [208] and preparation of nano-sized HA/polyamide (PA) biocomposites [209,210]. In certain cases, a mechanochemical route [211,212], emulsions [213–218], freeze-drying [219,220] and freeze-thawing techniques [221] or gel-templated mineralization [222] might be applied to produce $CaPO_4$-based biocomposites. Various fabrication procedures are well described elsewhere [22,37,199], where the interested readers are referred.

The interfacial bonding between the phases is an important issue of any $CaPO_4$/polymer biocomposite. A total of four types of mutual arrangements of nanodimensional particles to polymer chains have been classified by Kickelbick (Figure 1.1): (i) inorganic particles embedded in inorganic polymer, (ii) incorporation of particles by bonding to the polymer backbone, (iii) an interpenetrating network with chemical bonds, (iv) an inorganic–organic hybrid polymer [223]. If adhesion among the phases is poor, the mechanical properties of a biocomposite suffer. To solve the problem, various approaches have been already introduced. For example, a diisocyanate coupling agent was used to bind PEG/PBT (Polyactive™) block copolymers to HA filler particles. Using

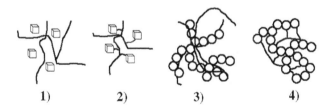

1)   2)   3)   4)

FIGURE 1.1   Four types of mutual arrangements of nano-sized particles to a polymer chain: (1) inorganic particles embedded in an inorganic polymer; (2) incorporation of particles by bonding to the polymer backbone; (3) interpenetrating network with chemical bonds; and (4) inorganic–organic hybrid polymer.

Source: Reprinted from Ref. [223] with permission.

surface-modified HA particles as a filler in a PEG/PBT matrix significantly improved the elastic modulus and strength of the polymer as compared to the polymers filled with ungrafted HA [194,224]. Another group used processing conditions to achieve a better adhesion of the filler to the matrix by pressing blends of varying PLLA and HA content at different temperatures and pressures [225]. The researchers found that maximum compressive strength was achieved at ~15 wt% of PLLA. Using blends with 20 wt% of PLLA, the authors also established that increasing the pressing temperature and pressure improved the mechanical properties. The former was explained by decrease in viscosity of the PLLA associated with a temperature increase, hence leading to improved wettability of HA particles. The latter was explained by increased compaction and penetration of pores at higher pressure, in conjunction with a greater fluidity of the polymer at higher temperatures. The combination of high pressures and temperatures was found to decrease porosity and guarantee a close apposition of a polymer to the particles, thereby improving the compressive strength [189] and fracture energy [226] of the biocomposites. The PLLA/HA biocomposite scaffolds were found to improve cell survival over plain PLLA scaffolds [227].

It is also possible to introduce porosity into $CaPO_4$-based biocomposites, which is advantageous for most applications as a bone-substitute material. The porosity facilitates migration of osteoblasts from surrounding bones to the implant site. Various material processing strategies to prepare composite scaffolds with interconnected porosity comprise thermally induced phase separation, solvent casting and particle leaching, solid freeform fabrication techniques, microsphere sintering and coating [123,228–231]. A supercritical gas foaming technique might be used as well [189,232,233].

1.4.1.1 Apatite-based Formulations

A biological apatite is known to be the major inorganic phase of mammalian calcified tissues [14,15]. Consequently, CDHA,

HA, carbonated apatite and, occasionally, fluorapatite (FA; all of them may be both pure and with dopants) have been applied to prepare biocomposites with other compounds, usually with the aim to improve the bioactivity. For example, polysulfone composed with HA can be used as a starting material for long-term implants [234–236]. Retrieved *in vivo*, HA/polysulfone biocomposite–coated samples from rabbit distal femurs demonstrated direct bone apposition to the coatings, as compared to the fibrous encapsulation that occurred when uncoated samples were used [234]. The resorption time of such biocomposites is a very important factor, which depends on polymer's microstructure and the presence of modifying phases [235].

Various apatite-containing biocomposites with polyvinyl alcohol (PVA) [221,237–242], polyvinyl alcohol phosphate (PVAP) [243] and several other polymeric components [244–255] have been already developed. Namely, PVA/CDHA biocomposite blocks were prepared by precipitation of CDHA in aqueous solutions of PVA [221]. An artificial cornea consisted of a porous nanosized HA/PVA hydrogel skirt and a transparent center of PVA hydrogel has been prepared as well. The results displayed a good biocompatibility and interlocking between artificial cornea and host tissues [237,238]. PVAP has been chosen as a polymer matrix, because its phosphate groups can act as a coupling/anchoring agent, which has a higher affinity toward the HA surface [245]. Greish and Brown developed HA/Ca poly(vinylphosphonate) biocomposites [247–249]. A template-driven nucleation and mineral growth process for the high-affinity integration of CDHA with polyhydroxyethyl methacrylate (PHEMA) hydrogel scaffold has been developed as well [252].

PEEK [133,134,256–262] and high-impact polystyrene [263,264] were also applied to create biocomposites with HA having a potential for clinical use in load-bearing applications. The study on reinforcing PEEK with thermally sprayed HA particles revealed that the mechanical properties increased monotonically with the reinforcement concentration, with a maximum value in the study of ~40% volume fraction of HA particles [256–258]. The reported ranges of stiffness within 2.8–16.0 GPa and strength within 45.5–69 MPa exceeded the lower values for human bone (7–30 GPa and 50–150 MPa, respectively) [257]. Modeling of the mechanical behavior of HA/PEEK biocomposites is available elsewhere [259].

Biodegradable poly(α-hydroxyesters) are well established in clinical medicine. Currently, they provide with a good choice when a suitable polymeric filler material is sought. For example, HA/PLGA formulations were developed which appeared to possess a cellular compatibility suitable for bone tissue regeneration [265–273]. Zhang and Ma seeded highly porous PLLA foams with HA particles in order to improve the osteoconductivity of polymer scaffolds for bone tissue engineering [193]. They pointed out that hydration of the foams prior to incubation in simulated body fluid increased the amount of carbonated CDHA material due to an increase of COOH and OH groups on the polymer surface, which apparently acted as nucleation sites for apatite. The mechanical properties of PLA/CaPO$_4$ biocomposites fabricated using different techniques, as well as the results of *in vitro* and *in vivo* experiments with them, are available in the literature [269].

On their own, poly(α-hydroxyesters), such as PGA and PLA, are known to degrade to acidic products (glycolic and lactic acids, respectively) that both catalyze polymer degradation and cause inflammatory reactions of the surrounding tissues [274]. Thus, in biocomposites of poly(α-hydroxyesters) with CaPO$_4$, the presence of slightly basic compounds (HA, TTCP) to some extent neutralizes the acid molecules, provides with a weak pH-buffering effect at the polymer surface and, therefore, more or less compensates these drawbacks [119,269,275–277]. However, additives of even more basic chemicals (*e.g.*, CaO, CaCO$_3$) might be necessary [123,277–279]. Extensive cell culture experiments on pH-stabilized composites of PGA and carbonated apatite were reported, which later were supported by extensive *in vitro* pH studies [280]. A consequent development of this approach has led to designing of functionally graded composite skull implants consisting of polylactides, carbonated apatite and CaCO$_3$ [281,282]. Besides the pH-buffering effect, inclusion of CaPO$_4$ was found to modify both surface and bulk properties of the biodegradable poly(α-hydroxyesters) by increasing the hydrophilicity and water absorption of the polymer matrix, thus altering the scaffold degradation kinetics. For example, polymer biocomposites filled with HA particles was found to hydrolyze homogeneously due to water penetrating into interfacial regions [283].

Biocomposites of poly(α-hydroxyesters) with CaPO$_4$ are prepared mainly by incorporating the inorganic phase into a polymeric solution, followed by drying under vacuum. The resulting solid biocomposites might be shaped using different processing techniques. One can also prepare these biocomposites by mixing HA particles with L-lactide prior the polymerization [275] or by a combination of slip casting technique and hot pressing [284]; however, other production techniques are known [269,271,285]. The addition of a surfactant (*surf*ace *active agent*) might be useful to keep the suspension homogeneity [286]. Furthermore, HA/PLA [214,215] and HA/PLGA [216] microspheres might be prepared by a microemulsion technique. More complex formulations, such as carbonated FA/PLA [287] and PLGA/carbon nanotubes/HA [288], are also known. An interesting list of references, assigned to the different ways of preparing HA/poly(α-hydroxyesters) biodegradable composites, is available in publications by Durucan and Brown [289–291]. The authors prepared CDHA/PLA and CDHA/PLGA biocomposites by solvent casting technique with a subsequent hydrolysis of α-tricalcium phosphate (TCP) to CDHA in aqueous solutions. The presence of both polymers was found to inhibit α-TCP hydrolysis, when compared with that of single-phase α-TCP; what is more, the inhibiting effect of PLA exceeded that of PLGA [289–291]. The physical interactions between CaPO$_4$ and poly(α-hydroxyesters) might be easily seen in Figure 1.2 [291]. Another set of good pictures might be found in Ref. [51]. Nevertheless, it should not be forgotten that typically

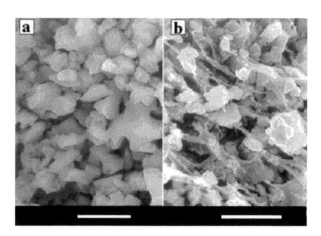

FIGURE 1.2   SEM micrographs of (a) α-TCP compact and (b) α-TCP/ PLGA biocomposite (bars = 5 μm).

Source: **Reprinted from Ref. [291] with permission.**

nonmelting-based routes lead to development of composites with lower mechanical performance, and many times require the use of toxic solvents and intensive hand labor [125].

The mechanical properties of poly(α-hydroxyesters) could be substantially improved by the addition of $CaPO_4$ [292,293]. Namely, CDHA/PLLA biocomposites of very high mechanical properties were developed [119], and fixation tools (screws and plates) made of these composites were manufactured and tested. These fixation tools revealed an easy handling and shaping according to the implant site geometry, total resorbability, good ability to bond directly to the bone tissue without interposed fibrous tissue, osteoconductivity, biocompatibility and high stiffness retainable for the period necessary to achieve bone union [283,285]. The initial bending strength of ~280 MPa exceeded that of cortical bone (120–210 MPa), while the modulus was as high as 12 GPa [119]. The strength could be maintained above 200 MPa up to 25 weeks in phosphate-buffered saline solution. These biocomposites could be obtained by precipitation from PLLA/

dichloromethane solutions, in which small particles of CaPO$_4$ were distributed [118,294]. Porous scaffolds of poly(D,L-lactic acid) (PDLLA) + HA [233,295,296] and PLGA + HA [297], as well as more complex formulations, such as PLA/ethyl cellulose/HA ones [298], were produced as well. On implantation into rabbit femora, a newly formed bone was observed, and biodegradation was significantly enhanced when compared to single-phase HA bioceramics. This might be due to a local release of lactic acid, which, in turn, dissolves HA. In other studies, PLA and PGA fibers were combined with porous HA scaffolds. Such reinforcement did not hinder bone ingrowth into the implants, which supported further development of such biocomposites as bone graft substitutes [29,269,270].

Blends (named as SEVA-C) of a copolymer of ethylene and vinyl alcohol (EVOH) with starch filled with 10–30 wt% HA have been fabricated to yield biocomposites with modulus up to ~7 GPa with a 30% HA loading [299–303]. The incorporation of bioactive fillers such as HA into SEVA-C aimed to assure the bioactive behavior of the composite and provide the necessary stiffness within the typical range of human cortical bone properties. These biocomposites exhibited a strong *in vitro* bioactivity that was supported by the polymer's water-uptake capability [304]. However, the reinforcement of SEVA-C by HA particles was found to affect the rheological behavior of the blend. A degradation model of these biocomposites has been developed [305].

Higher homologues poly(3-hydroxybutyrate), 3-PHB and poly(3-hydroxyvalerate) show almost no biodegradation. Nevertheless, biocomposites of these polymers with CaPO$_4$ showed a good biocompatibility both *in vitro* and *in vivo* [306–310]. Both bioactivity and mechanical properties of these biocomposites can be tailored by varying the volume percentage of CaPO$_4$. Similarly, biocomposites of poly(hydroxybutyrate-*co*-hydroxyvalerate) (PHBHV) with both HA and amorphous carbonated apatite (almost amorphous calcium phosphate (ACP)) appeared to have a promising potential for repair and replacement of damaged bones [311–314].

Along this line, PCL is used as a slowly biodegradable but well biocompatible polymer. PCL/HA and PCL/CDHA biocomposites have been already discussed as suitable materials for substitution, regeneration and repair of bone tissues [228,315–324]. For example, biocomposites were obtained by infiltration of ε-caprolactone monomer into porous apatite blocks and *in situ* polymerization [316]. The composites were found to be biodegradable and might be applied as cancellous or trabecular bone replacement material or for a cartilage regeneration. Both the mechanical performance and biocompatibility in osteoblast cell culture of PCL were shown to be strongly increased when HA was added [325]. Several preparation techniques of PCL/HA biocomposites are known [228,319]. For example, to make biocomposite fibers of PCL with nanodimensional HA, the desired amount of nanodimensional HA powder was dispersed in a solvent using magnetic stirrer followed by ultrasonication for 30 min. Then, PCL was dissolved in this suspension, followed by the solvent evaporation [326]. The opposite preparation order is also possible: PCL was initially dissolved in chloroform at room temperature (7%–10% w/v) and then HA (~10 μm particle size) was suspended in the solution, sonicated for 60 s, followed by the solvent evaporation [327] or salt leaching [328]. The mechanical properties obtained by this technique were about one third that of trabecular bone. In a comparative study, PCL and biological apatite were mixed in the ratio 19:1 in an extruder [329]. At the end of the preparation, the mixture was cooled in an atmosphere of nitrogen. The authors observed that the presence of biological apatite improved the modulus while concurrently increasing the hydrophilicity of the polymeric substrate. Besides, an increase in apatite concentration was found to increase both the modulus and yield stress of the composite, which indicated good interfacial interactions between the biological apatite and PCL. It was also observed that the presence of biological apatite stimulated osteoblasts attachment to the biomaterial and cell proliferation [329]. In another study, a PCL/HA biocomposite was prepared by blending in melt form at 120°C until the torque reached equilibrium in the rheometer that was attached to the blender [330]. Then, the sample was compression molded and cut into specimens of appropriate size for testing. It was observed that the composite containing 20 wt% HA had the highest strength [330]. However, a direct grafting of PCL on the surface of HA particles seems to be the most interesting preparation technique [315]. In another study, HA porous scaffolds were coated by a PCL/HA composite coating [331]. In this system, PCL, as a coating component, was able to improve the brittleness and low strength of the HA scaffolds, while the particles in the coating were to improve the osteoconductivity and bioactivity of the coating layer. More complex formulations, such as PDLLA/PCL/HA [332], PLLA/PCL/HA [333], FA-HA/PCL [334], magnetic PCL/Fe-doped HA [335] and supramolecular PCL/functionalized HA [336,337] biocomposites, have been prepared as well. Further details on both the PCL/HA biocomposites and the processing methodologies thereof might be found elsewhere [228,319,323].

To finalize this section, one should mention on HA biocomposites with other substances [338–341]. Some of them may exhibit interesting properties. Namely, it is worth mentioning on polymers with shape-memory characteristics [342]. Therefore, CaPO₄-based composites with such polymers appear to have the shape-memory properties as well [339–341]. Further details on HA/polymer biocomposites and hybrid biomaterials are available in other reviews [343,344].

1.4.1.2 TCP-based Formulations

Both α-TCP and β-TCP have a higher solubility than HA (Table 1.3). Besides, they are faster resorbed *in vivo* (however, there are some reports about a lack of TCP biodegradation after implantation in calvarial defects [345]). Therefore, α-TCP and β-TCP were widely used instead of apatites to prepare completely biodegradable biocomposites [346–367]. For example, a biodegradable and osteoconductive biocomposite made of β-TCP particles and gelatin was proposed [351]. This material was tested *in vivo* with good results. It was found to be biocompatible, osteoconductive and biodegradable with no need for a second surgical operation to remove the device after healing occurred. Both herbal extracts [352] and K_2HPO_4 [353] might be added to this formulation. Another research group prepared biocomposites of cross-linked gelatin with β-TCP, and both a good biocompatibility and bone formation on subcutaneous implantation in rats were found [354]. Yang et al. [358] extended this to porous (porosity ~75%) β-TCP/ gelatin biocomposites that also contained bone morphogenetic protein–4 (BMP-4). Furthermore, cell-compatible and posses-sive some osteoinductive properties porous β-TCP/alginate-gelatin hybrid scaffolds were prepared and successfully tested *in vitro* [355]. In addition, the $CaPO_4$ fillers were found to have a reinforcing effect [368]. More to the point, biocomposites of β-TCP with PLLA [294,346–349] and co-polyester lactide-*co*-glycolide-*co*-ε-caprolactone [350] were prepared. Although β-TCP was able to counter the acidic degradation of the polyester to some extent, it did not prevent a pH drop down to ~6. Nevertheless, implantation of this biocomposite in beagles' mandibular bones was successful [350]. α-TCP/gelatin formulations are known as well [361].

Based on a self-reinforcement concept, biocomposites of TCP with polylactides were prepared and studied using conventional mechanical testing [369]. Resorbable scaffolds were fabricated from such biocomposites [370]. Chitosan was also used as the matrix for the incorporation of β-TCP by a solid/liquid phase separation of the polymer solution and subsequent sublimation of the solvent. Due to complexation of the functional groups of chi-tosan with calcium ions of β-TCP, these biocomposites had high compressive modulus and strength [371]. PCL/β-TCP biocom-posites were developed in other studies [323,324,372–376], and their *in vitro* degradation behavior was systematically monitored by immersion in simulated body fluid at 37°C [374]. To extend this topic further, PCL/β-TCP biocomposites might be loaded by drugs [323,375].

An *in vitro* study with primary rat calvarial osteoblasts showed an increased cellular activity in the BMP-loaded samples [358]. Other researchers investigated BMP-2-loaded porous β-TCP/ gelatin biocomposites (porosity ~95%, average pore size 180– 200 μm) [377] and confirmed the precious study. A long-term implantation study of PDLLA/α-TCP composites in a loaded sheep implant model showed good results after 12 months but a strong osteolytic reaction after 24 months. This was ascribed to the almost complete dissolution of α-TCP to this time and an adverse reaction of the remaining PDLLA [378].

More complex CaPO$_4$-based formulations are known as well. For example, there is a biocomposite consisting of three interpenetrating networks: TCP, CDHA and PLGA [379]. First, a porous TCP network was produced by coating a PU foam by hydrolyzable α-TCP slurry. Then, a CDHA network was derived from self-setting CaPO$_4$ formulations filled in the porous TCP network. Finally, the remaining open-pore network in the CDHA/α-TCP structures was infiltrated with PLGA. This biocomposite consists of three phases with different degradation behaviors. It was postulated that bone would grow on the fastest degrading network of PLGA, while the remaining CaPO$_4$ phases would remain intact, thus maintaining their geometry and load-bearing capability [379]. In addition, PCL/TCP/boron nitride biocomposites were prepared as well [380].

1.4.1.3 Formulations based on Other Types of CaPO$_4$

The number of research publications devoted to formulations based on other types of CaPO$_4$ is substantially lesser than those devoted to apatites and TCP. Biphasic calcium phosphate (BCP), which is a solid composite of HA and β-TCP (however, similar formulations of HA and α-TCP, as well as of α-TCP and β-TCP, are known as well [381]) appears to be the most popular among the remaining types of $CaPO_4$. For example, collagen-coated BCP ceramics was studied, and the biocompatibility toward osteoblasts was found to increase on coating with collagen [382]. Another research group created porous PDLLA/BCP scaffolds and coated them with a hydrophilic PEG/vancomycin composite for both drug delivery purposes and surface modification [383]. More to the point, both PLGA/BCP [384,385] and PLLA/BCP [386] biocomposites were fabricated, and their cytotoxicity and fibroblast properties were found to be acceptable for natural bone tissue reparation, filling and augmentation [387,388]. Besides, PCL/BCP [389,390], poly(trimethylene carbonate) (PTMC)/BCP [391] and gelatin/BCP [392,393] biocomposites are known as well.

A choice of dicalcium phosphate dihydrate (DCPD)-based biocomposites of DCPD, albumin and duplex DNA was prepared by water/oil/water interfacial reaction method [213]. Core–shell-type DCPD/chitosan biocomposite fibers were prepared by a wet spinning method in another study [394]. The energy-dispersive X-ray spectroscopy analysis indicated that Ca and P atoms were mainly distributed on the outer layer of the composite fibers; however, a little amount of P atoms remained inside the fibers. This indicated that the composite fibers formed a unique core–shell structure with shell of $CaPO_4$ and core of chitosan [394]. A similar formulation was prepared for further applications in self-setting biocomposites [395]. Dicalcium phosphate anhydrous (DCPA)/ bovine serum albumin (BSA) biocomposites were synthesized through the coprecipitation of BSA on the nanodimensional particles of DCPA performed in ethanol [396], while DCPA/ ethyl cellulose ones were prepared by a sol–gel technique [397]. Nanodimensional DCPA was synthesized and incorporated into dental resins to form dental biocomposites [398–401], while porous DCPA/dextran/carboxymethylcellulose (CMC) nanocomposite scaffolds were prepared by lyophilization in a freeze-dryer [402]. Although, this is beyond the biomedical subject, it is interesting to mention that some DCPD/polymer composites could be used as proton conductors in battery devices [403,404]. Nothing has been reported on their biocompatibility, but perhaps, sometime, the improved formulations will be used to fabricate biocompatible batteries for implantable electronic devices.

To treat the consequences of dental caries, various ACP-based biocomposites and hybrid formulations for dental applications were developed [405,406]. Among them, there are rechargeable ones with sustained ion release and re-release, which were introduced in 2016 [407–410]. Besides, several ACP-based formulations were investigated as potential biocomposites for bone grafting [314,411–413] and drug delivery [414,415]. Namely, ACP/PPF biocomposites were prepared by *in situ* precipitation [412], while PHB/carbonated ACP and PHBHV/carbonated ACP biocomposites appeared to be well suited as a slowly biodegradable bone-substitute material [314].

Octacalcium phosphate (OCP)-based biocomposites with polymers are known as well. For example, granules of OCP were combined with gelatin, and the prepared composites were onlaid on rat calvaria. These composites were found to enhance bone augmentation through balanced osteoblastic and osteoclastic cellular activities [416]. Additional information on the biomedically relevant OCP-based formulations might be found in a topical review [417].

1.4.2 Biocomposites with Collagen

The main constituent of the bioorganic matrix of bones is type I collagen (Table 1.1) with molecules about 300 nm in length. The structural and biochemical properties of collagens have been widely investigated, and over 25 collagen subtypes have been identified [418,419]. All of them share the common characteristic of being composed for more than 50% by hydroxyproline, proline and glycine but differing for the remaining amino acidic composition. This peculiar composition is the cause of the triple helix conformation of collagen and its fibrillar arrangement. Such structure of collagen produces nanometric cavities where the inorganic phase nucleates and grows. This protein is easily degraded and resorbed by the body and allows good attachment to cells. Collagen alone is not effective as an osteoinductive material, but it becomes osteoconductive in combination with $CaPO_4$ [420]. Both collagen type I and HA were found to enhance osteoblast differentiation [421], but combined together, they were shown to accelerate osteogenesis. However, this tendency is not so straightforward: The data are available that implanted HA/collagen biocomposites enhanced regeneration of calvaria bone defects in young rats but postponed the regeneration of calvaria bone in aged rats [422]. Finally, the addition of $CaPO_4$ to collagen sheets was found to give a higher stability and an increased resistance to 3D swelling compared to the collagen reference [423]. Therefore, a bone analogue based on these two constituents should possess the remarkable properties.

The unique characteristics of bones are the spatial orientation between the nanodimentional crystals of biological apatite and collagen macromolecules at the nanoscale, where the crystals (about 50 nm length) are aligned parallel to the collagen fibrils, which is believed to be the source of the mechanical strength of bones [424]. The collagen molecules and the crystals of biological apatite assembled into mineralized fibrils are approximately 6 nm in diameter and 300 nm long. Although the complete mechanisms involved in the bone-building strategy are still unclear, the strengthening effect of nanodimentional crystals of biological apatite in calcified tissues might be explained by the fact that the collagen matrix is a load transfer medium and thus transfers the load to the intrinsically rigid inorganic crystals [14,15,19–21]. Furthermore, the crystals of biological apatite located in between tangled fibrils cross-link the fibers either through a mechanical interlocking or by forming calcium ion bridges, thus increasing deformation resistance of the collagenous fiber network [425].

When $CaPO_4$ are combined with collagen in a laboratory, the prepared biocomposites appear to be substantially different from natural bone tissue due to a lack of real interaction between the two components, that is, the interactions that are able to modify the intrinsic characteristics of the singular components themselves. The main characteristics of the route, by which the mineralized hard tissues are formed *in vivo*, are that the organic matrix is laid down first and the inorganic reinforcing phase grows within this organic matrix [14,15,20,21]. Although to date, neither the elegance of the biomineral assembly mechanisms nor the intricate composite nano-sized architectures have been duplicated by nonbiological methods, the best way to mimic bone is to copy the way it is formed, namely, by nucleation and growth of CDHA nano-sized crystals from a supersaturated solution both onto and within the collagen fibrils. Such syntheses were denoted as "biologically inspired," which means they reproduce an ordered pattern and an environment very similar to natural ones [426–428]. The biologically inspired biocomposites of collagen and CaPO$_4$ (mainly, apatites) for bone substitute have a long history [420,429–442] and started from the pioneering study by Banks et al., who grew CDHA on reconstituted calfskin collagen tapes in 1977 [443], followed by initial medical applications performed by other researchers in 1982 [444,445]. Such combinations were found to be bioactive, osteoconductive, osteoinductive [420,446–448], and in general, artificial grafts manufactured from this type of biocomposites are likely to behave similarly to bones and be of more use in surgery than those prepared from any other materials. Indeed, data are available on the superiority of CaPO$_4$/collagen biocomposite scaffolds over the artificial polymeric and CaPO$_4$ bioceramic scaffolds individually [449]. In addition, multiscale simulations of apatite/collagen composites were performed [450].

It has been found that CaPO$_4$ may be successfully precipitated onto a collagen substrate of whatever form or source [443,451,452]. However, adherence of CaPO$_4$ crystals to collagen did depend on how much the collagen had been denatured: The more fibrillar the collagen, the greater the attachment. Clarke et al. first reported the production of a biocomposite produced by precipitation of DCPD onto a collagen matrix with the aid of phosphorylated amino acids commonly associated with fracture sites [429]. Self-setting CDHA forming formulations (DCPD + TTCP) have been mixed with a collagen suspension, hydrated, and allowed to set. CDHA crystals were found to nucleate on the collagen fibril network, giving a material with the mechanical properties weaker than those reported for bone. More to the point, the prepared biocomposites were without the nanostructure similar to that of bone [430,453]. The oriented growth of OCP crystals on collagen was achieved by an experimental device in which Ca^{2+} and PO_4^{3-} ions diffused into a collagen disk from the opposite directions [453–455]. Unfortunately, these experiments were designed to simulate the mechanism of *in vivo* precipitation of biological apatite only; due to this reason, the mechanical properties of the biocomposites were not tested [456].

Conventionally, collagen/$CaPO_4$ biocomposites can be prepared by blending or mixing of collagen and $CaPO_4$, as well as by biomimetic methods [426–430, 440, 451, 456–467]. Tampieri et al. [428] produced and compared artificial bone-like tissue apatite/collagen biocomposites prepared using two different methodologies: (i) dispersion of apatite in a collagen aqueous suspension and then freeze-dried; and (ii) direct nucleation of an apatitic phase on assembling collagen fibrils. Biocomposites obtained using first way were similar to uncalcified natural collagen. The crystallite sizes were not uniform and were often aggregated and randomly distributed into the matrix, proving that there was no real interaction between apatite and collagen fibers. However, the second method allowed the direct nucleation of nano-sized crystals of apatite on self-assembled collagen fibers. In this case, the two components (CDHA and collagen) exhibited strong interactions, highlighted by several analysis techniques, which showed a complete analogy of the composite with calcified natural tissue [428]. Other production techniques are also possible. For example, using a polymer-induced liquid-precursor process, collagen/apatite biocomposites mimicking the nanostructure of bones, wherein nano-sized crystals of apatite were embedded within the collagen fibrils, were prepared [465]. More complicated formulations, such as a magnetite-enriched HA/collagen [468] and HA/collagen/PVA [469] biocomposites, have been developed as well. Recent investigations revealed that CaPO$_4$/collagen formulations might be printed by means of 3D printers [470].

In addition, collagen might be incorporated into various self-setting CaPO$_4$-based formulations [430,453,471–475]. Typically, a type I collagen sponge is presoaked in a PO$_4^{3-}$-containing highly basic aqueous solution and then is immersed into a Ca^{2+}-containing solution to allow mineral deposition. Also, collagen I fibers might be dissolved in acetic acid and then this solution is added to phosphoric acid, followed by a neutralization synthesis (performed at 25°C and solution pH within 9–10) between an aqueous suspension of Ca(OH)$_2$ and the H$_3$PO$_4$/collagen solution [426,427]. To ensure the quality of the final product, it is necessary to control the Ca/P ionic ratio in the reaction solution. One way to do this is to dissolve a commercial CaPO$_4$ in an acid; another one is to add Ca^{2+} and PO$_4^{3-}$ ions in a certain ratio to the solution and after that induce the reaction [476]. Biomimetically, one can achieve an oriented growth of CDHA crystals onto dissolved collagen fibrils in aqueous solutions via a self-organization mechanism [461]. More to the point, collagen might be first dispersed in an acidic solution, followed by the addition of calcium and orthophosphate ions, and then coprecipitation of collagen and CDHA might be induced by either increasing the solution pH or adding mixing agents. Although it resulted in biocomposites with poor mechanical properties, pressing of the apatite/collagen mixtures at 40°C under 200 MPa for several days is also known [477]. Attempts have been performed for a computer simulation of apatite/collagen composite formation process [478]. It is interesting to note that such biocomposites were found to possess some piezoelectric properties [479].

As the majority of the collagen/HA biocomposites are conventionally processed by anchoring micron-sized HA particles into collagen matrix, it makes quite difficult to obtain a uniform and homogeneous composite graft. Besides, such biocomposites have inadequate mechanical properties; over and above, the proper pore sizes have not been achieved either. Furthermore, microcrystalline HA, which is in contrast to nanocrystalline bone apatite, might take a longer time to be remodeled into a new bone tissue on the implantation. In addition, some of the biocomposites exhibited very poor mechanical properties, probably due to a lack of strong interfacial bonding between the constituents. Furthermore, in all blended composites, the crystallite sizes of $CaPO_4$ were not uniform, and the crystals were often aggregated and randomly distributed within a fibrous matrix of collagen. Therefore, no structural similarity to natural bone was obtained, and only a compositional similarity to that of natural bone was achieved. The aforementioned data clearly demonstrate that the chemical composition similar to bone is insufficient for manufacturing the proper grafts; both the mechanical properties and mimetic of the bone nanostructure are necessary to function as bone in recipient sites. There is a chance for improving osteointegration by reducing the grain size of HA crystals by activating of ultrafine apatite growth into the matrix. This may lead to enhance the mechanical properties and osteointegration with improved biological and biochemical affinity to the host bone. Besides, the porosity was found to have a positive influence on the ingrowth of the surrounding tissues into the pores of collagen/HA biocomposites [480,481].

Bovine collagen might be mixed with $CaPO_4$, and such biocomposites are marketed commercially as bone graft substitutes that can further be combined with bone marrow aspirated from the iliac crest of the site of the fracture. Bioimplant®, Bio-Oss Collagen®, Boneject®, Collagraft®, CollapAn®, Healos®, Integra Mozaik® and LitAr® are several examples of the commercially available $CaPO_4$/collagen grafts for the clinical use (Table 1.5). Application of these materials was compared with autografts for the management of acute fractures of long bones with defects, which had been stabilized by internal or external fixation [482,483]. These biocomposites

TABLE 1.5   A List of Known Commercially Produced CaPO$_4$-Containing Biocomposites and Hybrid Biomaterials

Composition	Trade Name and Producer (When Available)
HA embedded or suspended in a gel	NanoBone (Artoss, Germany)
	Nanogel (Teknimed, France)
	RADIESSE (Merz Aesthetics, Germany)
HA/collagen, CDHA/ collagen and/or carbonated apatite/ collagen	AUGMATRIX (Wright Medical Technology, TN, USA)
	Bioimplant (Connectbiopharm, Russia)
	Bio-Oss Collagen (Geitslich, Switzerland)
	Boneject (Koken, Japan)
	Collagraft (Zimmer and Collagen Corporation, USA)
	CollapAn (Intermedapatite, Russia)
	COLLAPAT (Symatese, France)
	G-Graft (Surgiwear, India)
	HAPCOL (Polystom, Russia)
	Healos (DePuy Spine, USA)
	LitAr (LitAr, Russia)
	OsteoTape (Impladent, NY, USA)
	RegenOss (JRI Orthopaedics, UK)
HA/sodium alginate	Bialgin (Biomed, Russia)
HA/poly-L-lactic acid	Biosteon (Biocomposites, UK)
	SuperFIXSORB30 (Takiron, Japan)
HA/polyethylene	HAPEX (Gyrus, TN, USA)
HA/CaSO$_4$	BioWrist Bone Void Filler (Skeletal Kinetics, CA, USA)
	CERAMENT (BONESUPPORT, Sweden)
	Hapset (LifeCore, MN, USA)
	PerOssal (aap Implantate, Germany)
β-TCP/CaSO$_4$	Genex (Biocomposites, UK)
β-TCP/poly-lactic acid	Bilok (Biocomposites, UK)
	Duosorb (SBM, France)
	Matryx® Interference Screws (Conmed, USA)
β-TCP/bone marrow aspirate	Induce (Skeletal Kinetics, CA, USA)
β-TCP/collagen	Integra Mozaik (Integra Orthobiologics, CA, USA)
β-TCP/rhPDGF-BB solution	AUGMENT Bone Graft (Wright Medical Group, TN, USA)

(Continued)

TABLE 1.5 (*Continued*)   A List of Known Commercially Produced CaPO$_4$-Containing Biocomposites and Hybrid Biomaterials

Composition	Trade Name and Producer (When Available)
BCP (HA + β-TCP)/ collagen	Allograft (Zimmer, IN, USA)
	Collacone max (botiss, Germany)
	Collagraft (Zimmer, IN, USA)
	Cross.Bone Matrix (Biotech Dental, France)
	Indost (Polystom, Russia)
	MasterGraft (Medtronic Sofamor Danek, TN, USA)
	MATRI BONE (Biom'Up, France)
	Without trade name (Medical Group, France)
BCP (HA + β-TCP)/ hydrogel	Eclipse (Citagenix, QC, Canada)
BCP (HA + β-TCP)/ polymer	In'Oss (Biomatlante, France)
	Hydros (Biomatlante, France)
	Osteotwin (Biomatlante, France)
BCP (HA + β-TCP)/ fibrin	TricOS (Baxter BioScience, France)
BCP (HA + β-TCP)/ silicon	FlexHA (Xomed, FL, USA)
DCPD/collagen	CopiOs Bone Void Filler (Zimmer, IN, USA)
DCPD + β-TCP/CaSO$_4$	PRO-DENSE (Wright Medical Group, TN, USA)
OCP/fibrin	FibroFor (BioNova, Russia)
Undisclosed CaPO$_4$ + biologics	i-FACTOR (Cerapedics, CO, USA)

are osteogenic, osteoinductive and osteoconductive; however, they lack the structural strength and require a harvest of the patient's bone marrow. OCP/collagen biocomposites have been investigated [484] and clinically tested [485].

Collagen sponges with an open porosity (30–100 μm) were prepared by a freeze-drying technique and then their surface was coated by a 10-μm layer of biomimetic apatite precipitated from simulated body fluid [486]. The researchers found a good *in vitro* performance with fibroblast cell culture. Other preparation techniques are also possible [487]. Collagen/HA microspheres or gel beads have been prepared in the intention of making injectable bone fillers [488–490]. Liao *et al.* succeeded in mimicking the bone structure by blending carbonated apatite with collagen [491]. A similar material (mineralized collagen) was implanted into femur of rats and excellent clinical results were observed after 12 weeks [492]. Collagen/HA biocomposites were prepared, and their mechanical performance was increased by cross-linking the collagen fibers with glutaraldehyde. A similar approach was selected to prepare HA/collagen microspheres (diameter ~5 μm) by a water–oil emulsion technique in which the surface was also cross-linked by glutaraldehyde [489]. This material showed a good *in vitro* performance with osteoblast cell culture. Porous (porosity level ~95% with interconnected pores of 50–100 μm) biocomposites of collagen (cross-linked with glutaraldehyde) and β-TCP have been prepared by a freeze-drying technique, followed by sublimation of the solvent; the biocomposites showed a good biocompatibility on implantation in the rabbit jaw [493].

Biocomposites of CaPO$_4$ with collagen were found to be useful for delivery of drugs, growth factors and other important biomolecules [432,475,494–496]. Namely, Gotterbarm *et al.* developed a two-layered collagen/β-TCP implant augmented with chondral inductive growth factors for repair of osteochondral defects in the trochlear groove of minipigs. This approach might be a new promising option for the treatment of deep osteochondral defects in joint surgery [495].

To conclude this part, one should note that biocomposites of apatites with collagen are a very hot topic of the research, and up until now, just a few articles are devoted to biocomposites of other CaPO$_4$ with collagen [458–460,495,497–500]. These biomaterials mimic natural bones to some extent, while their subsequent biological evaluation suggests that they are readily incorporated into the bone metabolism in a way similar to bone remodeling, instead of acting as permanent implant [445]. However, the performance of these biocomposites depends on the source of collagen from which it was processed. Several attempts have been made to simulate the collagen-HA interfacial behavior in real bone by means of cross-linking agents such as glutaraldehyde [451,489,493] with the purpose to improve the mechanical properties of these biocomposites. Unfortunately, a further progress in this direction is restricted by a high cost, difficulty to control cross-infection, a poor definition of commercial sources of collagens as well as by a lack of an appropriate technology to fabricate bone-resembling microstructures. Further details on the $CaPO_4$/collagen biocomposites might be found elsewhere [424,435,501].

1.4.3 Formulations with Other Bioorganic Compounds and/or Biological Macromolecules

The biggest practical problems with collagen type I are its cost and the poor definition of commercial sources of this material, which makes it difficult to follow up on well-controlled processing. Therefore, collagen type I can be replaced by other compounds. One should note that, besides collagen, both human and mammalian bodies contain dozen types of various bioorganic compounds, proteins and biological macromolecules. Therefore, the substantial amount of them potentially might be used to prepare biocomposites with $CaPO_4$. For example, a biologically strong adhesion (to prevent invasion of bacteria) between teeth and the surrounding epithelial tissues is attributed to a cell-adhesive protein, laminin [502]. In order to mimic the nature, a laminin/apatite biocomposite layer was successfully created on the surface of both titanium [503] and EVOH [504,505] using the biomimetic approach. A more complicated laminin/DNA/apatite biocomposite layer was found to be an efficient gene transfer system [506]. Further details on this subject are available in a topical review [507].

$CaPO_4$/gelatin biocomposites are widely investigated as potential bone replacement biomaterials [219,351–358,377,508–513]. For example, gelatin foams were successfully mechanically reinforced by HA and then cross-linked by a carbodiimide derivative [219]. Such foams were shown to be a good carrier for antibiotic tetracycline [509]. Several biocomposites of $CaPO_4$ with alginates have been prepared [355,427,514–518]. For example, porous HA/alginate composites based on hydrogels were prepared both biomimetically [427] and using a freeze-drying technique [514]. More complicated formulations have been developed as well [519,520].

Various biocomposites of CaPO$_4$ with chitosan [200,371, 394,411,521–532] and chitin [360,533–537] are also very popular. For example, a solution-based method was developed to combine HA powders with chitin, in which the ceramic particles were uniformly dispersed [533,534]. Unfortunately, it was difficult to obtain the uniform dispersions. The mechanical properties of the final biocomposites were not very good; due to a poor adhesion between the filler and the matrix, both the tensile strength and modulus were found to decrease with the increase in the HA amount. Microscopic examination revealed that HA particles were intervened between the polymer chains, weakening their interactions and decreasing the entire strength [533,534]. Other manufacturing techniques might be found in the aforementioned references; I just would like to mention on an interesting approach, in which an HA/chitosan biocomposite was produced by a hydrothermal process from natural CaCO$_3$/chitosan biocomposite of crab shells [526]. Similarly, HA/chitosan biocomposite was produced by a hydrothermal process from previously prepared DCPD/chitosan biocomposite [527]. Biocomposites of natural HA with chitosan were found to possess both a good hard tissue biocompatibility and an excellent osteoconductivity, which is suitable for artificial bone implants and frame materials of tissue engineering [523]. Data are available that addition of CaPO$_4$ into chitosan improved cell attachment and provided a higher cell proliferation and well-spread morphology when compared to chitosan alone [529]. More complex formulations, such as silk fiber–reinforced HA/chitosan [538] and HA/collagen/chitosan [539] biocomposites, have been studied as well. Besides biomedical applications, biocomposites of nano-sized HA with chitin/chitosan might be used for the removal of Fe(III) [540] and fluorides [541,542] from aqueous solutions.

Biocomposites of CDHA with water-soluble proteins, such as BSA, might be prepared by a precipitation method [543–546].

In such biocomposites, BSA is not strongly fixed to solid CDHA, which is useful for a sustained release. However, this is not the case if a water/oil/water interfacial reaction route has been used [213]. To extend this subject, inclusion of DNA into CDHA/BSA biocomposites was claimed [213,547–549]. Furthermore, biocomposites of an unspecified $CaPO_4$ with DNA [550,551] as well as those of nano-sized crystals of biomimetic apatite with C_{60} fullerene and Au-DNA nano-sized particles [552] were prepared as well.

Akashi and coworkers developed a procedure to prepare $CaPO_4$-based biocomposites by soaking hydrogels in solutions supersaturated by Ca^{2+} and PO_4^{3-} ions in order to precipitate CDHA in the hydrogels (up to 70% by weight of CDHA could be added to these biocomposites) [553]. This procedure was applied to chitosan; the 3D shape of the resulting biocomposite was controlled by the shape of the starting chitosan hydrogel [554]. Another research group developed biocomposites based on *in situ* $CaPO_4$ mineralization of self-assembled supramolecular hydrogels [555]. Other experimental approaches are also possible [556].

Various biocomposites of CDHA with glutamic and aspartic amino acids as well as poly-glutamic and poly-aspartic amino acids have been prepared and investigated [244,245,557–560]. These (poly)amino acids were quantitatively incorporated into CDHA crystals, provoking a reduction in the coherent length of the crystalline domains and decreasing the crystal sizes. The relative amounts of the (poly)amino acid content in the solid phase, determined through high-performance liquid chromatography analysis, increased with their concentration in solution up to a maximum of about 7.8 wt% for CDHA/aspartic acid and 4.3 wt% for CDHA/glutamic acid biocomposites. The small crystal dimensions, which implied a great surface area, and the presence of (poly)amino acids were suggested to be relevant for possible application of these biocomposites for hard tissues replacement [244,245,557–560].

Furthermore, BCP (HA + β-TCP)/agarose macroporous scaffolds with controlled and complete interconnection, high porosity, thoroughly open pores and tailored pore size were prepared for tissue engineering application [561,562]. Agarose, a biodegradable polymer, was selected as the organic matrix because it was a biocompatible hydrogel, which acted as gelling agent leading to strong gels and fast room temperature polymerization. Porous scaffolds with the designed architecture were manufactured by combining a low temperature shaping method with stereo-lithography and two drying techniques. The biocompatibility of this BCP/agarose system was tested with mouse L929 fibroblasts and human SAOS-2 (sarcoma osteogenic) osteoblasts during different colonization times [563].

Fibrin sealants are noncytotoxic, fully resorbable, biological matrices that simulate the final stages of a natural coagulation cascade, forming a structured fibrin clot similar to a physiological clot [564]. Biocomposites of CaPO$_4$ with fibrin sealants might develop the clinical applications of bone substitutes. The 3D mesh of fibrin sealant interpenetrates the macro- and microporous structure of CaPO$_4$ ceramics. The physical, chemical and biological properties of CaPO$_4$ bioceramics and the fibrin glue might be cumulated in biocomposites, suitable for preparation of advanced bone grafts [565–571].

Furthermore, there are biocomposites of CaPO$_4$ with bisphosphonates [572], silk fibroin [211,573–580], cellulose [581], chitosan + silk fibroin [582], chitosan + zein [583], chitosan derivatives [584], fibronectin [585], chondroitin sulfate [201,447,586], casein phosphopeptides [587], okra hydrocolloids [588], keratin [589], gellan gum [590] and graphene oxide/chitosan [591] hydrogels, amyloid fibrils [592], agarose [593], glycine [594] and vitamins [595]. Photopolymerizable formulations have been developed as well [596]. Besides, the reader's attention is pointed out to an interesting approach to crystallize CDHA inside poly(allylamine)/poly(styrene sulfonate) polyelectrolyte capsules resulting in empty biocomposite spheres of micron size. Depending on the amount of precipitated CDHA, the thickness of the shell of biocomposite spheres can be varied between 25 and 150 nm. These biocomposite capsules might find application as medical agents for bone repairing and catalytic microreactors [597].

An interesting phenomenon of fractal growth of FA/gelatin composite crystals (Figure 1.3) was achieved by diffusion of calcium- and orthophosphate + fluoride-containing solutions from the opposite sides into a tube filled with a gelatin gel [598–604]. The reasons of this phenomenon are not quite clear yet. Other types of $CaPO_4$-based composites, based on DCPD and OCP, were grown by the similar technique in an iota-carrageenan gel [605]. Up to now, nothing has yet been reported on a possible biomedical application of such unusual structural composites.

1.4.4 Injectable Bone Substitutes

With the development of minimally invasive surgical methods, for example, percutaneous surgery, directly injectable biomaterials are needed. The challenge is to place a biomaterial at the site of surgery by the least possible invasive method. In this regard, injectable bone substitute (IBS) appears to be a convenient

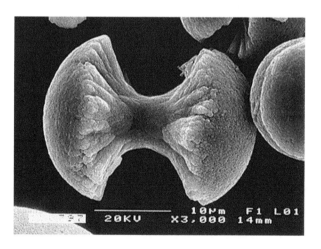

FIGURE 1.3   A biomimetically grown aggregate of FA that was crystallized in a gelatin matrix. Its shape can be explained and simulated by a fractal growth mechanism. Scale bar: 10 μm.

Source: Reprinted from Ref. [598] with permission.

alternative to solid bone-filling materials. They represent ready-to-use suspensions of CaPO$_4$ microspheres [606,607], nano-sized rods [608] or powder(s) in a liquid-carrier phase. However, the addition of other phases, such as calcium sulfate [609], is possible. Generally, IBSs appear like opaque viscous pastes with the rheological properties, sufficient to inject them into bone defects by means of surgical syringes and needles. Occasionally, their constituents may require to be mixed in the operating room, and in the latter case, it is sometimes possible to produce or combine the IBS with blood, bone marrow or platelet-rich plasma. Besides, IBS could be easily produced in a sterile stage. Their stable composition and mechanical properties are suitable for reproducibility of the biological response [610,611]. All types of IBS are divided into two major groups: self-setting formulations and those which do not set. The latter ones are described here.

IBS requires suitable rheological properties to ensure bonding and cohesion of the mineral phase *in situ* with good cell permeability. Usually, the necessary level of viscosity is created by the addition of suitable water-soluble polymers [92,217,612–621]. However, IBSs based on hydrogels are known as well [622–625]. Some of them possess self-gelling properties [625]. Therefore, the majority of CaPO$_4$-containing IBS formulations might be considered as a subgroup of CaPO$_4$/polymer biocomposites. For example, an IBS was described that it involved a silanized hydroxyethylcellulose carrier with BCP (HA + β-TCP). The suspension is liquid at pH within 10–12 but gels quickly at pH < 9 [614]. A polydioxanone-*co*-glycolide-based biocomposite reinforced with HA or β-TCP can be used as an injectable or moldable putty [615]. During the cross-linking reaction following injection, carbon dioxide is released allowing the formation of interconnected pores. Furthermore, HA/poly(L-lactide-*co*-ε-caprolactone) biocomposite microparticles were fabricated as an injectable scaffold via the Pickering emulsion route in the absence of any molecular surfactants. A stable injectable oil-in-water emulsion was obtained using water-dispersed HA nano-sized crystals as the particulate emulsifier and a dichloromethane solution of poly(L-lactide-*co*-ε-caprolactone) as an oil phase [217]. CaPO$_4$-containing IBS based on other (bio) organic compounds, such as CMC [618], oligo(poly(ethylene glycol) fumarate) [616,617] and chitosan + collagen [619], have been developed as well. In addition, photo-cross-linkable formulations are known [620].

Daculsi *et al.* developed viscous IBS biocomposites based on BCP (60% HA + 40% β-TCP) and 2% aqueous solution of hydroxypropylmethylcellulose (HPMC) that was said to be perfectly biocompatible, resorbable and easily fitted bone defects (due to an initial plasticity) [613,626–633]. The best ratio BCP/HPMC aqueous solution was found to be at ~65/35 w/w. To extend this subject further, IBS might be loaded by cells [634,635], radiopaque elements [636] or microparticles [637], as well as functionalized by nucleic acids [638]. Self-hardening formulations, based on Si-HPMC hydrogel, are known as well [634]. The list of the commercially available CaPO$_4$-based IBS formulations is presented in Table 1.6 [638]. Further details on IBS are available elsewhere [610,611].

1.5 INTERACTIONS AMONG THE PHASES IN CaPO$_4$-BASED FORMULATIONS

An important aspect that should be addressed in detail is a mutual interaction between CaPO$_4$ and other phases in biocomposites and hybrid biomaterials. In general, interactions among the phases in any composite can be either mechanical, when it results from radial compression forces exerted by the matrix on the filler particles (*e.g.*, developed during cooling due to thermal contraction), or chemical, when the reactivity of the filler toward the matrix has an important role. In the latter case, it is important to distinguish a physical interaction from chemical bonding [185]. According to Wypych [639], physical interaction is more or less temporary, implicating hydrogen bonding or van der Waals forces, whereas chemical bonding is stronger and more permanent, involving covalent bond formation. Thus, a chemical interfacial

TABLE 1.6   A List of Several Commercial Nonsetting CaPO$_4$-based IBS and Pastes with Indication of Producer, Product Name, Composition (When Available) and Form [638]

Producer	Product Name	Composition	Form
ApaTech (UK)	Actifuse™	HA, polymer and aqueous solution	Pre-mixed
	Actifuse™ Shape Actifuse™ ABX	Si-substituted CaPO$_4$ and a polymer	Pre-mixed
Baxter (US)	TricOs T TricOs	BCP (60% HA, 40% β-TCP) granules and Tissucol (fibrin glue)	To be mixed
Berkeley Advanced Biomaterials	Bi-Ostetic Putty	Not disclosed	Not disclosed
BioForm (US)	Calcium hydroxylapatite implant	HA powder embedded in a mixture of glycerine, water and CMC	Pre-mixed
Biomatlante (FR)	In'Oss™	BCP granules (60% HA, 40% β-TCP; 0.08–0.2 mm) and 2% HPMC	Pre-mixed
	MBCP Gel®	BCP granules (60% HA, 40% β-TCP; 0.08–0.2 mm) and 2% HPMC	Pre-mixed
	Hydr'Os	BCP granules (60% HA, 40% β-TCP; micro- and nano-sized particles) and saline solution	Pre-mixed
CERAMED (PT)	k-IBS®	BCP granules (75% HA, 25% β-TCP; 0.125–0.355 mm) and chitosan dissolved in PEG	Pre-mixed
	n-IBS®	Aqueous suspension of HA powders	Pre-mixed (*Continued*)

TABLE 1.6 (*Continued*) A List of Several Commercial Nonsetting CaPO$_4$-based IBS and Pastes with Indication of Producer, Product Name, Composition (When Available) and Form [638]

Producer	Product Name	Composition	Form
Degradable solutions (CH)	Easy graft™	β-TCP or BCP granules (0.45–1.0 mm) coated with 10-μm PLGA, *N*-methyl1-2-pyrrolydone	To be mixed
Dentsply (US)	Pepgen P-15® flow	HA (0.25–0.42 mm), P-15 peptide and aqueous Na hyaluronate solution	To be mixed
DePuy Spine (US)	Healos® Fx	HA (20–30%) and collagen	To be mixed
Fluidinova (P)	nanoXIM TCP	β-TCP (5 or 15%) and water	Pre-mixed
	nanoXIM HA	HA (5, 15, 30 or 40%) and water	Pre-mixed
Integra LifeSciences (US)	Mozaik Osteoconductive Scaffold	β-TCP (80%) and type 1 collagen (20%)	To be mixed
Mathys Ltd (CH)	Ceros® Putty/cyclOS® Putty	β-TCP granules (0.125–0.71 mm; 94%) and recombinant Na hyaluronate powder (6%)	To be mixed
Medtronic (US)	Mastergraft®	BCP (85% HA, 15% β-TCP) and bovine collagen	To be mixed
Merz Aesthetics (GER)	RADIESSE®	HA particles suspended in a gel	Pre-mixed
Osartis/AAP (GER)	Ostim®	Nanocrystalline HA (35%) and water (65%)	Pre-mixed
Smith & Nephew (US)	JAXTCP	β-TCP granules and an aqueous solution of 1.75% CMC and 10% glycerol	To be mixed
Stryker (US)	Calstrux™	β-TCP granules and CMC	To be mixed
Teknimed (FR)	Nanogel	HA (100–200 nm) (30%) and water (70%)	Pre-mixed
Therics (US)	Therigraft™ Putty	β-TCP granules and polymer	Pre-mixed
Zimmer (US)	Collagraft	BCP granules (65% HA, 35% β-TCP; 0.5–1.0 mm), bovine collagen and bone marrow aspirate	To be mixed

bond among the phases is preferred to achieve a higher strength of a composite. The magnitude of the interfacial bond among the phases determines how well a weak matrix transmits stress to the strong fibers. However, while a bond among the matrix and reinforcements must exist for the purpose of stress transfer, it should not be so strong that it prevents toughening mechanisms, such as debonding and fiber pullout.

There is still doubt as to the exact bonding mechanism among bone minerals (biological apatite) and bioorganics (collagen), which undoubtedly plays a critical role in determining the mechanical properties of bones. Namely, bone minerals are not directly bonded to collagen but through noncollagenous proteins that make up ~3% of bones (Table 1.1) and provide with active sites for biomineralization and cellular attachment [22]. In bones, the interfacial bonding forces are mainly ionic bonds, hydrogen bonds and hydrophobic interactions, which give the bones the unique composite behavior [291]. There is an opinion that opposite to bones, there is no sign of chemical bonding among the phases in conventional CaPO$_4$/collagen biocomposites, probably due to a lack of suitable interfacial bonding during mixing [476]. However, this is not the case for phosphorylated collagens [463]. Readers skilled in computer modeling are forwarded to simulations of the interactions between collagen peptides and HA surfaces [640] as well as between three polymers (PE, PA and PLA) and HA surfaces [641], respectively.

To study possible interactions among the phases, Fourier-transformed infrared (FTIR) spectra of some CaPO$_4$-based biocomposites and collagen films were collected and transformed into absorption spectra using the Kramers–Kronig equation to demonstrate energy shifts of residues on the apatite/collagen interface. After comparing FTIR spectra of biocomposites and collagen films in detail, red shifts of the absorption bands for C–O bonds were observed in the spectra of the biocomposites. These red shifts were described as a decrease in bonding energies of C–O bonds and assumed to be caused by an interaction with Ca^{2+} ions located on the surfaces of apatite nano-sized crystals [461]. Another proof of a chemical interaction between apatite and collagen was also evaluated in FTIR spectra of CDHA/collagen biocomposites, in which a shift of the band corresponding to $-COO^-$ stretching from 1340 to 1337 cm^{-1} was observed [426,427]. More to the point, nucleation of apatite crystals onto collagen through a chemical interaction with carboxylate groups of collagen macromolecules has been reported [642–644].

FTIR spectroscopy seems to be the major tool to study a possible chemical bonding among the phases in $CaPO_4$-based biocomposites and hybrid biomaterials [178,209,243,250,251,346,412,427,463,511,512,552,582,624,645–652]. For example, the characteristic bands at 2918, 2850 and 1472 cm^{-1} for the hydrocarbon backbone of PE appeared to have zero shift in an HA/PE biocomposite. However, in the case of PA, several FTIR bands indicated that the polar groups shifted apparently: the bands at 3304, 1273 and 692 cm^{-1} derived from stretching of N–H, stretching of C–N–H and vibrating of N–H moved to 3306, 1275 and 690 cm^{-1}, respectively, in the HA/PA biocomposites. Furthermore, both stretching (3568 cm^{-1}) and vibrating (692 cm^{-1}) modes of hydroxide in HA moved to 3570 and 690 cm^{-1} in the HA/PA biocomposites, respectively, indicating the formation of hydrogen bonds. Besides, bands at 1094 and 1031 cm^{-1} of PO_4 modes also shifted to 1093 and 1033 cm^{-1} in HA/PA biocomposites. The band shift in a fingerprint area indicated that the hydroxide and orthophosphate on the surface of HA might interact with plentiful carboxyl and amino groups of PA through nucleophilic addition [178]. Comparable conclusions were made for CDHA/alginate [427], ACP/PPF [412], HA/maleic anhydride [251], HA/carboxylated PU [651] and β-TCP/PLLA [346] biocomposites, in which weak chemical bonds were considered to form between Ca^{2+} ions located on the HA, CDHA, ACP or β-TCP surface, respectively, and slightly polarized O atoms of C=O bonds in the surrounding bioorganic compounds. The data obtained suggested that crystallization of $CaPO_4$ in chitosan-containing solutions was substantially modulated by a chemical interaction of the components; apparently, a part of calcium was captured by chitosan and did not participate in the formation of the main mineral phase [650].

Except FTIR spectroscopy, other measurement techniques are also able to show some evidences of a chemical interaction among the phases in $CaPO_4$-based biocomposites and hybrid biomaterials [243,346,646–654]. For example, for nano-sized crystals of CDHA/alendronate, such evidences were observed by thermogravimetric analysis: Derivative of thermogravimetric analysis plots of the crystals appeared to be quite different from those obtained from mechanical mixtures of CDHA and calcium alendronate with similar compositions [653]. In the case of biocomposites of nano-sized HA with PA, a hydrogen bonding among the phases was detected by differential scanning calorimetry technique [647]. One more example comprises application of the dynamic mechanical analysis to investigate softening mechanism of β-TCP/PLLA biocomposites [346]. As to biocomposites of nano-sized HA with PVAP, some indirect evidences of a chemical bonding among the phases were found by X-ray diffraction and thermogravimetric analysis [243]. A strong structural correlation between the orientation of FA crystallites and gelatin within the FA/gelatin composite spheres was discovered that indicated a substantial reorganization of the macromolecular matrix within the area of a growing aggregate [598]. An inverse gas chromatography at infinite dilution was found to be able to provide some data on thermodynamic interactions between $CaPO_4$ and PLLA [654]. In addition, chemical interactions between HA and organic molecules have been elucidated using *ab initio* calculation methods [655].

By means of the X-ray photo-electronic spectroscopy technique, binding energies of Ca, P and O atoms were found to have some differences between the surface P–OH groups of HA and C=O groups of PDLLA [647]. The interaction and adhesion between $CaPO_4$ fillers and respective matrixes have a significant effect on the properties of particulate-filled-reinforced materials, being essential to transfer the load among the phases and thus improve the mechanical performance of the biocomposites [250]. However, for a substantial amount of the aforementioned formulations, the interactions among the phases is mechanical in nature. This is because the matrix often consists of compounds with no functional groups or unsaturated bonds, which can form ionic complexes with the constituents of $CaPO_4$. Obviously, less coupling exists between nonpolar polymers and $CaPO_4$ ceramic particles. Therefore, polymers with functional groups pendant to the polymer backbone, which can act as sites for bridging to $CaPO_4$, are more promising in this respect [291].

In order to influence the interactions among the phases, various supplementary reagents are applied. Namely, if the primary effect of a processing additive is to increase the interaction between the phases, such additives can be regarded as coupling agents [656]. These agents establish chemical bridges between the matrix and the fillers, promoting adhesion among the phases. In many cases, their effect is not unique; for example, it might also influence rheology of the composites [185]. In the case of $CaPO_4$, a hexamethylene diisocyanate coupling agent was used to bind PEG/PBT (Polyactive™) block copolymers [194] and other polymers [645] to HA filler particles. Thermogravimetric and infrared analyses demonstrated that the polymers were chemically bonded to the HA particles through the isocyanate groups, making it a suitable approach to improve the adhesion [645]. Other researchers used glutaraldehyde as a cross-linked reagent [358,420,451,489,493,657]. In addition, the interfacial bonding among $CaPO_4$ and other components might be induced by silanes [170,171,194,303,658–663], zirconates [185,303,305,664–666], titanates [185,333,665,667], alkaline pretreatment [573,575], polyacrylic acid [668] and some other chemicals. Structural modifications of the polymeric matrices, for instance, with the introduction of acrylic acid [152,170,171,194], have also proved to be effective methods. For example, application of polyacids as a bonding agent for HA/Polyactive composites caused the surface-modified HA particles to maintain better contact with the polymer at fracture and improved mechanical properties [194]. The use of titanate and zirconate coupling agents appeared to be very dependent on the molding technique employed [185]. Silane-coupled HA powders were tested before applying them as fillers in biodegradable composites. This treatment allowed HA withstanding the attack of aqueous solutions without impairing overall bioactivity [659–663]. Besides, a chemically modified reinforcement phase–matrix interface was found to improve the mechanical properties of the biocomposites. The examples include chemically coupled HA/PE [170,171], chemically formed HA/Ca poly(vinylphosphonate) [247] and PLA/HA fibers [144]. These biocomposites are able to consume a large amount of energy in the fracture.

The action of some coupling agents was found to combine two distinct mechanisms: (i) cross-linking of the polymeric matrix (valid for zirconate and titanate coupling agents) and (ii) improvement of the interfacial interactions among the major phases of the biocomposites. This interfacial adhesion improvement appeared to be much dependent on the chemical nature (pH and type of metallic center) of the coupling agents [303]. Several works claimed that silanes did interact with HA [170,235,659–661]. It was shown that a silicon-containing interphase existed between HA and PE, which promoted the chemical adhesion between the HA particles and the polymer. A silane-coupling agent also facilitated penetration of PE into cavities of individual HA particles, which resulted in enhanced mechanical interlocking at the matrix-reinforcement interface [170,171].

In addition to the aforementioned, the surface of CaPO₄ might be modified as well [666–676]. An interesting approach for HA surface modification was described [675]. First, *in situ* synthesis of surface thiol-functionalized HA (HA-SH) was realized by adding 3-mercaptopropionic acid during hydrothermal synthesis of HA. This was followed by grafting polymerization of ethylene glycol methacrylate phosphate by radical chain transfer generating the sulfur-centered radicals on the HA surfaces, which initiated the surface grafting polymerization of ethylene glycol methacrylate phosphate [675]. In certain cases, the surface functionalization of $CaPO_4$ particles was found to decrease the bacterial adherence on their surface [676]. Other examples might be found in the literature [664–676]. In general, the purpose of surface modifying is not only to guarantee the even distribution of $CaPO_4$ particles at a high loading level in the matrix but also to prevent or delay the debonding process of $CaPO_4$ particles from the matrix. Obviously, all surface modifiers must satisfy several biomedical requirements, such as no toxicity, good biocompatibility and no changes in the biological or physicochemical properties of the fillers.

The addition of adhesion-promoting agents might be an alternative to improve the interaction between the fillers and the matrix. For example, Morita *et al.* incorporated 4-methacryloyloxyethyl trimellitic anhydride to promote adhesion of the polymer to HA [677]. In another study, a phosphoric ester was added to the liquid component of the formulation [678]. Both the strength and the affinity index of biocomposites were found to increase, probably due to the effects of copolymerization.

Possible interactions between BCP and HPMC have been investigated in IBS composites [628,629,679]. After mixing, there was a decrease in the mean diameter of BCP granules, and this influenced the viscosity of the paste. Dissolution of grain boundaries of β-TCP crystals and precipitation of CDHA on HA crystal surface were found during the interaction. Both phenomena were responsible for the observed granulometric changes [628,629]; however, within the sensitivity of the employed measurement techniques, no chemical bonding between BCP and HPMC was detected [679].

A coprecipitation technique was used to prepare CDHA/chitosan biocomposites [521]. Growth of CDHA crystals was inhibited by organic acids with more than two carboxyl groups, which strongly bind to CDHA surfaces via COO–Ca bonds. Transmission electron microscopy images revealed that CDHA formed elliptic aggregates with chemical interactions (probably coordination bond) between Ca on its surface and amino groups of chitosan; the nano-sized crystals of CDHA were found to align along the chitosan molecules, with the amino groups working as the nucleation sites [521]. A chemical bond between the phases was presumed in PCL/HA composites, prepared by the grafting technique [315]; unfortunately, no strong experimental evidences were provided. In another study, CDHA/poly(α-hydroxyester) composites were prepared by a low temperature chemical route [289]. In that study, pre-composite structures were prepared by combining α-TCP with PLA, PLGA and copolymers thereof. The final biocomposite was achieved by in situ hydrolysis of α-TCP to CDHA performed at 56°C in either solvent cast or pressed pre-composites. This transformation occurred without any chemical reaction between the polymer and CaPO$_4$, as it was determined by FTIR spectroscopy [289].

1.6 BIOACTIVITY AND BIODEGRADATION OF CaPO$_4$/POLYMER FORMULATIONS

The continuous degradation of an implant causes a gradual load transfer to the healing tissue, preventing stress-shielding atrophy and stimulates the healing and remodeling of bones. Some requirements must be fulfilled by the ideal prosthetic biodegradable materials, such as biocompatibility, adequate initial strength and stiffness, retention of mechanical properties throughout sufficient time to assure its biofunctionality and nontoxicity of the degradation by-products [125]. In most cases, bioactivity (*i.e.*, ability of bonding to bones) of biologically relevant CaPO$_4$ reinforced by other materials is lower than that of pure CaPO$_4$ [680].

In general, both bioactivity and biodegradability of any biocomposite and/or hybrid biomaterial are determined by the same properties of the constituents. Both processes are very multifactorial because during implantation, the surface of any graft contacts with biological fluids and, shortly afterward, is colonized by cells. Much more biology, than chemistry and material science altogether, is involved into these very complex processes, and many specific details still remain unknown. In addition, biodegradation of all components of biocomposites occurs simultaneously, and the obtained by-products might influence both the entire process and biodegradation of each component. For example, in the case of biocomposites prepared from polyesters and TCP, hydrolysis reactions of the ester bonds, acid dissociation of the carboxylic end groups, dissolution of TCP and buffering reactions by the dissolved phosphate ions occur simultaneously [681–684]. In such cases, basic TCP buffer the acidic degradation products of polyesters, thus reducing autocatalysis and delaying polymer degradation. This is why both pH and mass drops occurred at earlier degradation time points for the pure polymer samples than for the corresponding composites. However, this is not always the case. Namely, studies are available, in which the presence of $CaPO_4$ did not have an effect on the degradation rate of the polymer matrix [685–687]. Therefore, to simplify the task, biodegradation of the individual components should be considered independently. Namely, an *in vitro* biodegradation of the biologically relevant $CaPO_4$ might be described by their chemical dissolution in slightly acidic media (they are almost insoluble in alkaline solutions [74,75]), which, in the case of CDHA, might be described as a sequence of four successive chemical equations (1.1)–(1.4) [688,689]:

$$Ca_{10-x}(HPO_4)_x(PO_4)_{6-x}(OH)_{2-x} + (2-x)H^+$$
$$= Ca_{10-x}(HPO_4)_x(PO_4)_{6-x}(H_2O)_{2-x}^{(2-x)+} \tag{1.1}$$

$$Ca_{10-x}(HPO_4)_x(PO_4)_{6-x}(H_2O)_{2-x}^{(2-x)+}$$
$$= 3Ca_3(PO_4)_2 + (1-x)Ca^{2+} + (2-x)H_2O \tag{1.2}$$

$$Ca_3(PO_4)_2 + 2H^+ = Ca^{2+} + 2CaHPO_4 \tag{1.3}$$

$$CaHPO_4 + H^+ = Ca^{2+} + H_2PO_4^- \tag{1.4}$$

Biodegradability of polymers generally depends on the following factors: (i) chemical stability of the polymer backbone;

(ii) hydrophobicity of the monomer; (iii) morphology of the polymer; (iv) initial molecular weight; (v) fabrication processes; (vi) geometry of the implant; and (vii) properties of the scaffold such as porosity and pore diameter [228]. A summary on degradation of PLA and PGA, as well as that of SEVA-C, is available in the literature [125, p. 798 and p. 803, respectively], where the interested readers are referred.

Concerning *in vivo* studies, biodegradation of HA/PLLA and CDHA/PLLA biocomposite rods in subcutis and medullary cavities of rabbits were investigated mechanically and histologically; the degradation was found to be faster for the case of using uncalcined CDHA instead of calcined HA [690]. In a more detailed study, new bone formation was detected at two weeks after implantation, especially for formulations with a high HA content [691]. More to the point, a direct contact between bones and these composites without intervening fibrous tissue was detected in this case [691,692]. Both SEVA-C and SEVA-C/HA biocomposites were found to exhibit a noncytotoxic behavior [693,694], inducing a satisfactory tissue response when implanted as shown by *in vivo* studies [695]. Furthermore, SEVA-C/HA biocomposites induced a positive response on osteoblast-like cells to what concerned cell adhesion and proliferation [693]. An *in vivo* study on biodegradation of microspheres (PLGA, gelatin and PTMC were used)/CaPO$_4$ biocomposites revealed that they exhibited microsphere degradation after 12 weeks of subcutaneous implantation, which was accompanied by compression strength decreasing [695]. Interestingly that the amount of CaPO$_4$ in biocomposites was found to have a greater effect on the early stages of osteoblast behavior (cell attachment and proliferation) rather than the immediate and late stages (proliferation and differentiation) [696].

Both *in vitro* (the samples were immersed into 1% trypsin/phosphate-buffered saline solution at 37°C) and *in vivo* (implantation of samples into the posterolateral lumbar spine of rabbits) biodegradation were investigated for nano-sized HA/collagen/PLA biocomposites [697]. The results demonstrated that weight loss increased continuously *in vitro* with a reduction in mass of ~20% after 4 weeks. During the experimental period *in vitro*, a relative rate of reduction of the three components in this material was shown to differ greatly: collagen decreased the fastest, from 40% by weight to ~20% in the composite; HA content increased from 45% to ~60%; while the amount of PLA changed a little. *In vivo*, the collagen/HA ratio appeared to be slightly higher near the transverse process than in the central part of the inter-transverse process [697]. Hasegawa *et al.* [698] performed *in vivo* study, spanning over a period of 5–7 years, on high-strength HA/ PLLA biocomposite rods for the internal fixation of bone frac-tures. In that work, both uncalcined CDHA and calcined HA were used as reinforcing phases in PLLA matrix. Those composites were implanted in the femurs of 25 rabbits. It was found that the implanted materials were resorbed after 6 years of implantation. The presence of remodeled bone and trabecular bone bonding was the significant outcome. These data clearly demonstrate a biodeg-radation independence of various components of biocomposites.

1.7 CONCLUSIONS

All types of calcified tissues of humans and mammals appear to possess a complex hierarchical biocomposite structure. Their mechanical properties are outstanding (considering weak constituents from which they are assembled) and far beyond those that can be achieved using the same synthetic materials with pres-ent technologies. This is because biological organisms produce biocomposites that are organized in terms of both composition and structure, containing both brittle $CaPO_4$ and ductile bio-organic components in very complex structures, hierarchically organized at the nano, micro and meso levels. In addition, the cal-cified tissues are always multifunctional: for example, bone pro-vides structural support for the body plus blood cell formation. The third defining characteristic of biological systems, in contrast with current synthetic systems, is their self-healing ability, which is nearly universal in nature. These complex structures, which have risen from millions of years of evolution, inspire material scientists in the design of novel biomaterials [395].

Obviously, no single-phase biomaterial is able to provide all the essential features of bones and/or other calcified tissues, and therefore, there is a great need to engineer multiphase biomaterials (biocomposites) with a structure and composition mimicking those of natural bones. The properties of polymers such as low melting points, a good blend compatibility, and acceptable rheological properties enable their use by almost any polymer processing technology to manufacture and manipulate it into a large range of scaffolds for bone tissue engineering applications. Nevertheless, the majority of polymers suffer from some shortcomings such as slow degradation rates, poor mechanical properties, and low cell adhesion. The integration of composite techniques to develop high-strength and bioactive CaPO$_4$/polymer biocomposites and hybrid biomaterials with controllable degradation rates making them promising biomaterials for bone tissue engineering applications due to their osteoconductivity, biodegradability, and high mechanical strength.

The studies summarized in this book have shown that the proper combination of a ductile matrix with a brittle, hard, and bioactive CaPO$_4$ filler offers many advantages for biomedical applications. Namely, the desirable properties of some components can compensate for a poor mechanical behavior of CaPO$_4$ bioceramics, while, in turn, the desirable bioactive properties of CaPO$_4$ improve those of other phases, thus expanding the possible application of each material within the body [69,70]. However, the reviewed literature clearly indicates that among possible types of CaPO$_4$/polymer biocomposites and hybrid biomaterials only simple, complex and graded ones as well as fibrous, laminar, and particulate ones have been investigated. Presumably, a future progress in this subject will require concentrating efforts on elaboration and development of both hierarchical and hybrid biocomposites. Furthermore, following the modern tendency of tissue engineering, a novel generation of CaPO$_4$/polymer biocomposites and hybrid biomaterials should also contain a biological living part.

To conclude, the future of the $CaPO_4$/polymer biocomposites and hybrid biomaterials is now directly dependent on the formation of multidisciplinary teams composed of experts but primarily experts ready to collaborate in close collaboration with others and thus be able to deal efficiently with the complexity of the human organism. The physical chemistries of solids, solid surfaces, polymer dispersion, and solutions, as well as material–cell interactions, are among the phenomena to be tackled. Furthermore, much work remains to be done on a long way from a laboratory to clinics, and the success depends on the effective cooperation of clinicians, chemists, biologists, bioengineers and materials scientists. It is anticipated that a continued development and optimization of $CaPO_4$-based biocomposites and hybrid biomaterials with polymers will ensure a new generation of biomimetic and functional bone grafts is made available to patients.

ABBREVIATIONS

BMP	bone morphogenetic protein
BSA	bovine serum albumin
CMC	carboxymethylcellulose
EVOH	a copolymer of ethylene and vinyl alcohol
HDPE	high-density polyethylene
HPMC	hydroxypropylmethylcellulose
IBS	injectable bone substitute
PA	polyamide
PAA	polyacrylic acid
PBT	polybutylene terephthalate
PCL	poly(ε-caprolactone)
PDLLA	poly(D,L-lactic acid)
PE	polyethylene
PEEK	polyetheretherketone
PEG	polyethylene glycol

PGA   polyglycolic acid
PHB   polyhydroxybutyrate
PHBHV   poly(hydroxybutyrate-*co*-hydroxyvalerate)
PHEMA   polyhydroxyethyl methacrylate
PLA   polylactic acid
PLGA   poly(lactic-*co*-glycolic) acid
PLGC   co-polyester lactide-*co*-glycolide-*co*-ε-caprolactone
PLLA   poly(ʟ-lactic acid)
PMMA   polymethyl methacrylate
PP   polypropylene
PPF   poly(propylene-*co*-fumarate)
PTMC   poly(trimethylene carbonate)
PU   polyurethane
PVA   polyvinyl alcohol
PVAP   polyvinyl alcohol phosphate
SEVA-C   a blend of EVOH with starch

REFERENCES

1. Chau A.M.T., Mobbs R.J., Bone graft substitutes in anterior cervical discectomy and fusion. *Eur. Spine J.*, (2009), 18, 449–464.
2. Kaveh K., Ibrahim R., Bakar M.Z.A., Ibrahim T.A., Bone grafting and bone graft substitutes. *J. Anim. Vet. Adv.*, (2010), 9, 1055–1067.
3. Shibuya N., Jupiter D.C., Bone graft substitute: allograft and xenograft. *Clin. Podiatr. Med. Surg.*, (2015), 32, 21–34.
4. Conway J.D., Autograft and nonunions: morbidity with intramedullary bone graft versus iliac crest bone graft. *Orthop. Clin. North Am.*, (2010), 41, 75–84.
5. Li S., Chen Y., Lin Z., Cui W., Zhao J., Su W., A systematic review of randomized controlled clinical trials comparing hamstring autografts versus bone-patellar tendon-bone autografts for the reconstruction of the anterior cruciate ligament. *Arch. Orthop. Trauma Surg.*, (2012), 132, 1287–1297.
6. Keller E.E., Triplett W.W., Iliac crest bone grafting: review of 160 consecutive cases. *J. Oral Maxillofac. Surg.*, (1987), 45, 11–14.
7. Schaaf H., Lendeckel S., Howaldt H.P., Streckbein P., Donor site morbidity after bone harvesting from the anterior iliac crest. *Oral Surg. Oral Med. Oral Pathol. Oral Radiol. Endod.*, (2010), 109, 52–58.
8. Carlsen A., Gorst-Rasmussen A., Jensen T., Donor site morbidity associated with autogenous bone harvesting from the ascending mandibular ramus. *Implant Dent.*, (2013), 22, 503–506.

9. Qvick L.M., Ritter C.A., Mutty C.E., Rohrbacher B.J., Buyea C.M., Anders M.J., Donor site morbidity with reamer-irrigator-aspirator (RIA) use for autogenous bone graft harvesting in a single centre 204 case series. *Injury*, (2013), 44, 1263–1269.

10. Li Z., Kawashita M., Current progress in inorganic artificial biomaterials. *J. Artif. Organ.*, (2011), 14, 163–170.

11. Bojar W., Kucharska M., Ciach T., Koperski Ł., Jastrzębski Z., Szałwiński M., Bone regeneration potential of the new chitosan-based alloplastic biomaterial. *J. Biomater. Appl.*, (2014), 28, 1060–1068.

12. Panchbhavi V.K., Synthetic bone grafting in foot and ankle surgery. *Foot Ankle Clin.*, (2010), 15, 559–576.

13. Dinopoulos H., Dimitriou R., Giannoudis P.V., Bone graft substitutes: what are the options? *Surgeon*, (2012), 10, 230–239.

14. Weiner S., Wagner H.D., The material bone: structure-mechanical function relations. *Ann. Rev. Mater. Sci.*, (1998), 28, 271–298.

15. Rey C., Combes C., Drouet C., Glimcher M.J., Bone mineral: update on chemical composition and structure. *Osteoporos. Int.*, (2009), 20, 1013–1021.

16. Dorozhkin S.V., *Calcium Orthophosphates: Applications in Nature, Biology, and Medicine*, Pan Stanford, Singapore, 2012, p. 854.

17. Dorozhkin S.V., *Calcium Orthophosphate-Based Bioceramics and Biocomposites*, Wiley-VCH: Weinheim, Germany, 2016, p. 405.

18. Burr D.B., The contribution of the organic matrix to bone's material properties. *Bone*, (2002), 31, 8–11.

19. Fratzl P., Gupta H.S., Paschalis E.P., Roschger P., Structure and mechanical quality of the collagen-mineral nano-composite in bone. *J. Mater. Chem.*, (2004), 14, 2115–2123.

20. Olszta M.J., Cheng X.G., Jee S.S., Kumar B.R., Kim Y.Y., Kaufman M.J., Douglas E.P., Gower L.B., Bone structure and formation: a new perspective. *Mater. Sci. Eng. R*, (2007), 58, 77–116.

21. Fonseca H., Moreira-Gonçalves D., Coriolano H.J.A., Duarte J.A., Bone quality: the determinants of bone strength and fragility. *Sports Med.*, (2014), 44, 37–53.

22. Murugan R., Ramakrishna S., Development of nanocomposites for bone grafting. *Compos. Sci. Technol.*, (2005), 65, 2385–2406.

23. Suchanek W., Yoshimura M., Processing and properties of hydroxyapatite-based biomaterials for use as hard tissue replacement implants. *J. Mater. Res.*, (1998), 13, 94–117

24. Vallet-Regi M., Arcos D., Nanostructured hybrid materials for bone tissue regeneration. *Curr. Nanosci.*, (2006), 2, 179–189.

25. Doblaré, M., Garcia J.M., Gómez M.J., Modelling bone tissue fracture and healing: a review. *Eng. Fract. Mech.*, (2004), 71, 1809–1840.

26. Vallet-Regi M., Revisiting ceramics for medical applications. *Dalton Trans.*, (2006), 5211–5220.

27. Pioletti D.P., Biomechanics in bone tissue engineering. *Comput. Methods Biomech. Biomed. Engin.*, (2010), 13, 837–846.

28. Huiskes R., Ruimerman R., van Lenthe H.G., Janssen J.D., Effects of mechanical forces on maintenance and adaptation of form in trabecular bone. *Nature*, (2000), 405, 704–706.

29. Boccaccini A.R., Blaker J.J., Bioactive composite materials for tissue engineering scaffolds. *Expert Rev. Med. Dev.*, (2005), 2, 303–317.

30. Hutmacher D.W., Schantz J.T., Lam C.X.F., Tan K.C., Lim T.C., State of the art and future directions of scaffold-based bone engineering from a biomaterials perspective. *J. Tissue Eng. Regen. Med.*, (2007), 1, 245–260.

31. Guarino V., Causa F., Ambrosio L., Bioactive scaffolds for bone and ligament tissue. *Expert Rev. Med. Dev.*, (2007), 4, 405–418.

32. Yunos D.M., Bretcanu O., Boccaccini A.R., Polymer-bioceramic — composites for tissue engineering scaffolds. *J. Mater. Sci.*, (2008), 43, 4433–4442.

33. Zhao H.X., Progress of study on drug-loaded chitosan/hydroxyapatite composite in bone tissue engineering. *J. Funct. Mater.*, (2014), 45, 13006–13012+13020.

34. Hench L.L., Polak J.M., Third-generation biomedical materials. *Science*, (2002), 295, 1014–1017.

35. Mathijsen A., *Nieuwe Wijze van Aanwending van het Gips-Verband bij Beenbreuken*, J.B. van Loghem: Haarlem, Netherlands, 1852, p. 21.

36. Dreesman H., Über Knochenplombierung. *Beitr. Klin. Chir.*, (1892), 9, 804–810.

37. Wang M., Developing bioactive composite materials for tissue replacement. *Biomaterials*, (2003), 24, 2133–2151.

38. https://en.wikipedia.org/wiki/Composite_material (assessed in June 2018).

39. Gibson R.F., A review of recent research on mechanics of multifunctional composite materials and structures. *Compos. Struct.*, (2010), 92, 2793–2810.

40. Evans S.L., Gregson P.J., Composite technology in load-bearing orthopaedic implants. *Biomaterials*, (1998), 19, 1329–1342.

41. Wan Y.Z., Hong L., Jia S.R., Huang Y., Zhu Y., Wang Y.L., Jiang H.J., Synthesis and characterization of hydroxyapatite-bacterial cellulose nanocomposites. *Compos. Sci. Technol.*, (2006), 66, 1825–1832.

42. Wan Y.Z., Huang Y., Yuan C.D., Raman S., Zhu Y., Jiang H.J., He F., Gao C., Biomimetic synthesis of hydroxyapatite/bacterial cellulose nanocomposites for biomedical applications. *Mater. Sci. Eng. C*, (2007), 27, 855–864.

43. Ohtsuki C., Kamitakahara M., Miyazaki T., Coating bone-like apatite onto organic substrates using solutions mimicking body fluid. *J. Tissue Eng. Regen. Med.*, (2007), 1, 33–38.

44. Oyane A., Development of apatite-based composites by a biomimetic process for biomedical applications. *J. Ceram. Soc. Jpn.*, (2010), 118, 77–81.

45. Dorozhkin S.V., Calcium orthophosphate deposits: preparation, properties and biomedical applications. *Mater. Sci. Eng. C*, (2015), 55, 272–326.
46. Surmenev R.A., Surmeneva M.A., Ivanova A.A., Significance of calcium phosphate coatings for the enhancement of new bone osteogenesis – a review. *Acta Biomater.*, (2014), 10, 557–579.
47. Dorozhkin S.V., Calcium orthophosphate coatings on magnesium and its biodegradable alloys. *Acta Biomater.*, (2014), 10, 2919–2934.
48. Zhao J., Guo L.Y., Yang X.B., Weng J., Preparation of bioactive porous HA/PCL composite scaffolds. *Appl. Surf. Sci.*, (2008), 255, 2942–2946.
49. Dorozhkin S., Ajaal T., Toughening of porous bioceramic scaffolds by bioresorbable polymeric coatings. *Proc. Inst. Mech. Eng. H*, (2009), 223, 459–470.
50. Woo A.S., Jang J.L., Liberman R.F., Weinzweig J., Creation of a vascularized composite graft with acellular dermal matrix and hydroxyapatite. *Plast. Reconstr. Surg.*, (2010), 125, 1661–1669.
51. Zhao J., Duan K., Zhang J.W., Lu X., Weng J., The influence of polymer concentrations on the structure and mechanical properties of porous polycaprolactone-coated hydroxyapatite scaffolds. *Appl. Surf. Sci.*, (2010), 256, 4586–4590.
52. Dong J., Uemura T., Kojima H., Kikuchi M., Tanaka J., Tateishi T., Application of low-pressure system to sustain *in vivo* bone formation in osteoblast/porous hydroxyapatite composite. *Mater. Sci. Eng. C*, (2001), 17, 37–43.
53. Zerbo I.R., Bronckers A.L.J.J., de Lange G., Burger E.H., Localisation of osteogenic and osteoclastic cells in porous β-tricalcium phosphate particles used for human maxillary sinus floor elevation. *Biomaterials*, (2005), 26, 1445–1451.
54. Mikán, J., Villamil M., Montes T., Carretero C., Bernal C., Torres M.L., Zakaria F.A., Porcine model for hybrid material of carbonated apatite and osteoprogenitor cells. *Mater. Res. Innov.*, (2009), 13, 323–326.
55. Oe K., Miwa M., Nagamune K., Sakai Y., Lee S.Y., Niikura T., Iwakura T., Hasegawa T., Shibanuma N., Hata Y., Kuroda R., Kurosaka M., Nondestructive evaluation of cell numbers in bone marrow stromal cell/β-tricalcium phosphate composites using ultrasound. *Tissue Eng. C*, (2010), 16, 347–353.
56. Krout A., Wen H.B., Hippensteel E., Li P., A hybrid coating of biomimetic apatite and osteocalcin. *J. Biomed. Mater. Res. A*, (2005), 73A, 377–387.
57. Kundu B., Soundrapandian C., Nandi S.K., Mukherjee P., Dandapat N., Roy S., Datta B.K., Mandal T.K., Basu D., Bhattacharya R.N., Development of new localized drug delivery system based on ceftriaxone-sulbactam composite drug impregnated porous hydroxyapatite: a systematic approach for *in vitro* and *in vivo* animal trial. *Pharm. Res.*, (2010), 27, 1659–1676.

58. Kickelbick G. (ed.), *Hybrid Materials. Synthesis, Characterization, and Applications*, Wiley-VCH Verlag: Weinheim, Germany, 2007, p. 498.
59. Matthews F.L., Rawlings R.D., *Composite Materials: Engineering and Science*, CRC Press: Boca Raton, FL, 2000, p. 480.
60. Xia Z., Riester L., Curtin W.A., Li H., Sheldon B.W., Liang J., Chang B., Xu J.M., Direct observation of toughening mechanisms in carbon nanotube ceramic matrix composites. *Acta Mater.*, (2004), 52, 931–944.
61. Tavares M.I.B., Ferreira O., Preto M., Miguez E., Soares I.L., da Silva E.P., Evaluation of composites miscibility by low field NMR. *Int. J. Polym. Mater.*, (2007), 56, 1113–1118.
62. Kiran E., Polymer miscibility, phase separation, morphological modifications and polymorphic transformations in dense fluids. *J. Supercrit. Fluids*, (2009), 47, 466–483.
63. Šupová, M., Problem of hydroxyapatite dispersion in polymer matrices: a review. *J. Mater. Sci. Mater. Med.*, (2009), 20, 1201–1213.
64. Böstman O., Pihlajamäki H., Clinical biocompatibility of biodegradable orthopaedic implants for internal fixation: a review. *Biomaterials*, (2000), 21, 2615–2621.
65. John M.J., Thomas S., Biofibres and biocomposites. *Carbohydr. Polym.*, (2008), 71, 343–364.
66. Rea S.M., Bonfield W., Biocomposites for medical applications. *J. Aust. Ceram. Soc.*, (2004), 40, 43–57.
67. Tanner K.E., Bioactive ceramic-reinforced composites for bone augmentation. *J. R. Soc. Interface*, (2010), 7, S541–S557.
68. Gravitis Y.A., Tééyaér, R.E., Kallavus U.L., Andersons B.A., Ozol'-Kalnin V.G., Kokorevich A.G., Érin'sh P.P., Veveris G.P., Biocomposite structure of wood cell membranes and their destruction by explosive autohydrolysis. *Mech. Compos. Mater.*, (1987), 22, 721–725.
69. Bernard S.L., Picha G.J., The use of coralline hydroxyapatite in a 'biocomposite' free flap. *Plast. Reconstr. Surg.*, (1991), 87, 96–107.
70. Dorozhkin S.V., Calcium orthophosphates and human beings. A historical perspective from the 1770s until 1940. *Biomatter*, (2012), 2, 53–70.
71. Dorozhkin S.V. A detailed history of calcium orthophosphates from 1770s till 1950. *Mater. Sci. Eng. C*, (2013), 33, 3085–3110.
72. Hing K.A., Bioceramic bone graft substitutes: influence of porosity and chemistry. *Int. J. Appl. Ceram. Technol.*, (2005), 2, 184–199.
73. Naqshbandi A.R., Sopyan I., Gunawan, Development of porous calcium phosphate bioceramics for bone implant applications: a review. *Rec. Pat. Mater. Sci.*, (2013), 6, 238–252.
74. LeGeros R.Z., *Calcium Phosphates in Oral Biology and Medicine. Monographs in Oral Science*, Myers H.M. (ed.), Karger: Basel, Switzerland, 1991, vol. 15, p. 201.

75. Elliott J.C., *Structure and Chemistry of the Apatites and Other Calcium Orthophosphates, Studies in Inorganic Chemistry*, Elsevier: Amsterdam, Netherlands, 1994, vol. 18, p. 389.

76. Amjad Z. (ed.), *Calcium Phosphates in Biological and Industrial Systems*. Kluwer: Boston, MA, 1997, p. 529.

77. Heimann R.B. (ed.), *Calcium Phosphate: Structure, Synthesis, Properties, and Applications*, Nova Science: New York, 2012, p. 498.

78. Gshalaev V.S., Demirchan A.C. (eds), *Hydroxyapatite: Synthesis, Properties and Applications*. Nova Science: New York, 2012, p. 477.

79. Carraher C.E., Jr. *Introduction to Polymer Chemistry*, 2nd edn, CRC Press: Boca Raton, FL, 2010, p. 534.

80. Young R.J., Lovell P.A., *Introduction to Polymers*, 3rd edn, CRC Press: Boca Raton, FL, 2011, p. 688.

81. Thomson R.C., Ak S., Yaszemski M.J., Mikos A.G., Polymer scaffold processing. In: *Principles of Tissue Engineering*, Academic Press: New York, 2000, pp. 251–262.

82. Ramakrishna S., Mayer J., Wintermantel E., Leong K.W., Biomedical applications of polymer-composite materials: a review. *Compos. Sci. Technol.*, (2001), 61, 1189–1224.

83. Shastri V.P. Non-degradable biocompatible polymers in medicine: past, present and future. *Curr. Pharm. Biotechnol.*, (2003), 4, 331–337.

84. Chen H., Yuan L., Song W., Wu Z., Li D., Biocompatible polymer materials: role of protein-surface interactions. *Prog. Polym. Sci.*, (2008), 33, 1059–1087.

85. Tanaka M., Sato K., Kitakami E., Kobayashi S., Hoshiba T., Fukushima K., Design of biocompatible and biodegradable polymers based on intermediate water concept. *Polymer J.*, (2015), 47, 114–121.

86. Lanza R.P., Hayes J.L., Chick W.L., Encapsulated cell technology. *Nature Biotechnol.*, (1996), 14, 1107–1111.

87. Shukla S.C., Singh A., Pandey A.K., Mishra A., Review on production and medical applications of ε-polylysine. *Biochem. Eng. J.*, (2012), 65, 70–81.

88. Agrawal C.M., Ray R.B., Biodegradable polymeric scaffolds for musculoskeletal tissue engineering. *J. Biomed. Mater. Res.*, (2001), 55, 141–150.

89. Kweon H., Yoo M., Park I., Kim T., Lee H., Lee S., Oh J., Akaike T., Cho C., A novel degradable polycaprolactone network for tissue engineering. *Biomaterials*, (2003), 24, 801–808.

90. Wang Y.C., Zhang P.H., Electrospun absorbable polycaprolactone (PCL) scaffolds for medical applications. *Adv. Mater. Res.*, (2014), 906, 221–225.

91. Sartori S., Chiono V., Tonda-Turo C., Mattu C., Gianluca C., Biomimetic polyurethanes in nano and regenerative medicine. *J. Mater. Chem. B*, (2014), 2, 5128–5144.

92. Temenoff J.S., Mikos A.G., Injectable biodegradable materials for orthopedic tissue engineering. *Biomaterials*, (2000), 21, 2405–2412.

93. Behravesh E., Yasko A.W., Engel P.S., Mikos A.G., Synthetic biodegradable polymers for orthopaedic applications. *Clin. Orthop. Rel. Res.*, (1999), 367S, S118–S125.

94. Lewandrowski K.U., Gresser J.D., Wise D.L., White R.L., Trantolo D.J., Osteoconductivity of an injectable and bioresorbable poly(propyleneglycol-*co*-fumaric acid) bone cement. *Biomaterials*, (2000), 21, 293–298.

95. Lee K.W., Wang S., Fox B.C., Ritman E.L., Yaszemski M.J., Lu L. Poly(propylene fumarate) bone tissue engineering scaffold fabrication using stereolithography: effects of resin formulations and laser parameters. *Biomacromolecules*, (2007), 8, 1077–1084.

96. Xu J., Feng E., Song J., Renaissance of aliphatic polycarbonates: new techniques and biomedical applications. *J. Appl. Polym. Sci.* (2014), 131, 39822 (16 pages).

97. Boland E.D., Coleman B.D., Barnes C.P., Simpson D.G., Wnek G.E., Bowlin G.L., Electrospinning polydioxanone for biomedical applications. *Acta Biomater.*, (2005), 1, 115–123.

98. Gilbert J.L., Acrylics in biomedical engineering. In: *Encyclopedia of Materials: Science and Technology*, Elsevier: Amsterdam, Netherlands, 2001, pp. 11–18.

99. Frazer R.Q., Byron R.T., Osborne P.B., West K.P., PMMA: an essential material in medicine and dentistry. *J. Long-Term Eff. Med. Implants*, (2005), 15, 629–639.

100. Li Y.W., Leong J.C., Y., Lu W.W., Luk K.D, K., Cheung K.M.C., Chiu K.Y., Chow S.P. A novel injectable bioactive bone cement for spinal surgery: a developmental and preclinical study. *J. Biomed. Mater. Res.*, (2000), 52, 164–170.

101. Mckellop H., Shen F., Lu B., Campbell P., Salovey R., Development of an extremely wear resistant UHMW polyethylene for total hip replacements. *J. Orthop. Res.*, (1999), 17, 157–167.

102. Kurtz S.M., Muratoglu O.K., Evans M., Edidin A.A., Advances in the processing, sterilization and crosslinking of ultra-high molecular weight polyethylene for total joint arthroplasty. *Biomaterials*, (1999), 20, 1659–1688.

103. Laurencin C.T., Ambrosio M.A., Borden M.D., Cooper J.A., Jr. Tissue engineering: orthopedic applications. *Ann. Rev. Biomed. Eng.*, (1999), 1, 19–46.

104. Meijer G.J., Cune M.S., van Dooren M., de Putter C., van Blitterswijk C.A., A comparative study of flexible (Polyactive™) versus rigid (hydroxylapatite) permucosal dental implants. I. Clinical aspects. *J. Oral Rehabil.*, (1997), 24, 85–92.

105. Meijer G.J., Dalmeijer R.A., de Putter C., van Blitterswijk C.A., A comparative study of flexible (Polyactive™) versus rigid (hydroxylapatite) permucosal dental implants. II. Histological aspects. *J. Oral Rehabil.*, (1997), 24, 93–101.

106. Waris E., Ashammakhi N., Lehtimäki M., Tulamo R.M., Törmälä, P., Kellomäki M., Konttinen Y.T. Long-term bone tissue reaction to polyethylene oxide/polybutylene terephthalate copolymer (Polyactive®) in metacarpophalangeal joint reconstruction. *Biomaterials*, (2008), 29, 2509–2515.

107. Svensson A., Nicklasson E., Harrah T., Panilaitis B., Kaplan D.L., Brittberg M., Gatenholm P., Bacterial cellulose as a potential scaffold for tissue engineering of cartilage. *Biomaterials*, (2005), 26, 419–431.

108. Rampinelli G., di Landro L., Fujii T., Characterization of biomaterials based on microfibrillated cellulose with different modifications. *J. Reinf. Plast. Compos.*, (2010), 29, 1793–1803.

109. Granja P.L., Barbosa M.A., Pouysége L., de Jéso B., Rouais F., Baquuey C., Cellulose phosphates as biomaterials. Mineralization of chemically modified regenerated cellulose hydrogels. *J. Mater. Sci.*, (2001), 36, 2163–2172.

110. Granja P.L., Jéso B.D., Bareille R., Rouais F., Baquey C., Barbosa M.A., Cellulose phosphates as biomaterials. *In vitro* biocompatibility studies. *React. Funct. Polym.*, (2006), 66, 728–739.

111. Thomas V., Dean D.R., Vohra Y.K., Nanostructured biomaterials for regenerative medicine. *Curr. Nanosci.*, (2006), 2, 155–177.

112. Dee K.C., Bizios R. Mini-review: proactive biomaterials and bone tissue engineering. *Biotechnol. Bioeng.*, (1996), 50, 438–442.

113. Ashammakhi N., Rokkanen P., Absorbable polyglycolide devices in trauma and bone surgery. *Biomaterials*, (1997), 18, 3–9.

114. Boyan B., Lohmann C., Somers A., Neiderauer G., Wozney J., Dean D., Carnes D., Schwartz Z., Potential of porous poly-D,L-lactide-*co*-glycolide particles as a carrier for recombinant human bone morphogenetic protein-2 during osteoinduction *in vivo*. *J. Biomed. Mater. Res.*, (1999), 46, 51–59.

115. Hollinger J.O., Leong K., Poly(α-hydroxyacids): carriers for bone morphogenetic proteins. *Biomaterials*, (1996), 17, 187–194.

116. Griffith L.G., Polymeric biomaterials. *Acta Mater.*, (2000), 48, 263–277.

117. Peter S.J., Miller M.J., Yasko A.W., Yaszemski M.J., Mikos A.G., Polymer concepts in tissue engineering. *J. Biomed. Mater. Res.*, (1998), 43, 422–427.

118. Ishuang S.L., Payne R.G., Yaszemski M.J., Aufdemorte T.B., Bizios R., Mikos A.G., Osteoblast migration on poly(α-hydroxy esters). *Biotechnol. Bioeng.*, (1996), 50, 443–451.

119. Shikinami Y., Okuno M., Bioresorbable devices made of forged composites of hydroxyapatite (HA) particles and poly-L-lactide (PLLA): Part I. Basic characteristics. *Biomaterials*, (1999), 20, 859–877.

120. Khor E., Lim L.Y., Implantable applications of chitin and chitosan. *Biomaterials*, (2003), 24, 2339–2349.

121. di Martino A., Sittinger M., Risbud M.V. Chitosan: a versatile biopolymer for orthopaedic tissue-engineering. *Biomaterials*, (2005), 26, 5983–5990.

122. Piskin E., Bölgen N., Egri S., Isoglu I.A., Electrospun matrices made of poly(α-hydroxy acids) for medical use. *Nanomedicine*, (2007), 2, 441–457.

123. Rezwana K., Chena Q.Z., Blakera J.J., Boccaccini A.R., Biodegradable and bioactive porous polymer/inorganic composite scaffolds for bone tissue engineering. *Biomaterials*, (2006), 27, 3413–3431.

124. Seal B.L., Otero T.C., Panitch A., Polymeric biomaterials for tissue and organ regeneration. *Mater. Sci. Eng. R*, (2001), 34, 147–230.

125. Mano J.F., Sousa R.A., Boesel L.F., Neves N.M., Reis R.L. Bioinert, biodegradable and injectable polymeric matrix composites for hard tissue replacement: state of the art and recent developments. *Compos. Sci. Technol.*, (2004), 64, 789–817.

126. Middleton J., Tipton A., Synthetic biodegradable polymers as orthopedic devices. *Biomaterials*, (2000), 21, 2335–2346.

127. Coombes A.G., Meikle M.C., Resorbable synthetic polymers as replacements for bone graft. *Clin. Mater.*, (2004), 17, 35–67.

128. de las Heras Alarcón, C., Pennadam S., Alexander C., Stimuli responsive polymers for biomedical applications. *Chem. Soc. Rev.*, (2005), 34, 276–285.

129. Kohane D.S., Langer R., Polymeric biomaterials in tissue engineering. *Pediatric Res.*, (2008), 63, 487–491.

130. Okada M., Chemical syntheses of biodegradable polymers. *Prog. Polym. Sci.*, (2002), 27, 87–133.

131. Peterson G.I., Dobrynin A.V., Becker M.L., Biodegradable shape memory polymers in medicine. *Adv. Healthcare Mater.*, (2017), 6, 1700694.

132. Jordan J., Jacob K.I., Tannenbaum R., Sharaf M.A., Jasiuk I., Experimental trends in polymer nanocomposites – a review. *Mater. Sci. Eng. A*, (2005), 393, 1–11.

133. Converse G.L., Yue W., Roeder R.K., Processing and tensile properties of hydroxyapatite-whisker-reinforced polyetheretherketone. *Biomaterials*, (2007), 28, 927–935.

134. Converse G.L., Roeder R.K., Tensile properties of hydroxyapatite whisker reinforced polyetheretherketone. *Mater. Res. Soc. Symp. Proc.*, (2005), 898, 44–49.

135. Choi W.Y., Kim H.E., Kim M.J., Kim U.C., Kim J.H., Koh Y.H., Production and characterization of calcium phosphate (CaP) whisker-reinforced poly(ε-caprolactone) composites as bone regenerative. *Mater. Sci. Eng. C*, (2010), 30, 1280–1284.

136. Zhang H., Darvell B.W., Failure and behavior in water of hydroxyapatite whisker-reinforced bis-GMA-based resin composites. *J. Mech. Behav. Biomed. Mater.*, (2012), 10, 39–47.

137. Liu F., Wang R., Cheng Y., Jiang X., Zhang Q., Zhu M., Polymer grafted hydroxyapatite whisker as a filler for dental composite resin with enhanced physical and mechanical properties. *Mater. Sci. Eng. C*, (2013), 33, 4994–5000.

76 ■ Calcium Orthophosphates with Polymers

138. Liu F.W., Bao S., Jin Y., Jiang X.Z., Zhu M.F., Novel bionic dental resin composite reinforced by hydroxyapatite whisker. *Mater. Res. Innov.* (2014), 18, S4854–S4858.
139. Nouri-Felekori M., Mesgar A.S.M., Mohammadi Z., Development of composite scaffolds in the system of gelatin – calcium phosphate whiskers/fibrous spherulites for bone tissue engineering. *Ceram. Int.*, (2015), 41, 6013–6019.
140. Watanabe T., Ban S., Ito T., Tsuruta S., Kawai T., Nakamura H., Biocompatibility of composite membrane consisting of oriented needle-like apatite and biodegradable copolymer with soft and hard tissues in rats. *Dental Mater. J.*, (2004), 23, 609–612.
141. Li H., Chen Y., Xie Y. Photo-crosslinking polymerization to prepare polyanhydride/needle-like hydroxyapatite biodegradable nanocomposite for orthopedic application. *Mater. Lett.*, (2003), 57, 2848–2854.
142. Nejati E., Firouzdor V., Eslaminejad M.B., Bagheri F. Needle-like nano hydroxyapatite/poly(L-lactide acid) composite scaffold for bone tissue engineering application. *Mater. Sci. Eng. C*, (2009), 29, 942–949.
143. Sun S.P., Wei M., Olson J.R., Shaw M.T., A modified pultrusion process for preparing composites reinforced with continuous fibers and aligned hydroxyapatite nano needles. *Polym. Composite*, (2015), 36, 931–938.
144. Kasuga T., Ota Y., Nogami M., Abe Y., Preparation and mechanical properties of polylactic acid composites containing hydroxyapatite fibers. *Biomaterials*, (2000), 22, 19–23.
145. Smith L. Ceramic-plastic material as a bone substitute. *Arch. Surg.*, (1963), 87, 653–661.
146. Bonfield W., Grynpas M.D., Tully A.E., Bowman J., Abram J., Hydroxyapatite reinforced polyethylene – a mechanically compatible implant material for bone replacement. *Biomaterials*, (1981), 2, 185–189.
147. Bonfield W., Bowman J., Grynpas M.D., Composite material for use in orthopaedics, *UK Patent* 8032647, (1981).
148. Bonfield W., Composites for bone replacement. *J. Biomed. Eng.*, (1988), 10, 522–526.
149. Guild F.J., Bonfield W., Predictive character of hydroxyapatite-polyethelene HAPEX™ composite. *Biomaterials*, (1993), 14, 985–993.
150. Huang J., di Silvio L., Wang M., Tanner K.E., Bonfield W., In vitro mechanical and biological assessment of hydroxyapatite-reinforced polyethylene composite. *J. Mater. Sci. Mater. Med.*, (1997), 8, 775–779.
151. Wang M., Joseph R., Bonfield W., Hydroxyapatite-polyethylene composites for bone substitution: effect of ceramic particle size and morphology. *Biomaterials*, (1998), 19, 2357–2366.
152. Ladizesky N.H., Ward I.M., Bonfield W., Hydroxyapatite/high-performance polyethylene fiber composites for high load bearing bone replacement materials. *J. Appl. Polym. Sci.*, (1997), 65, 1865–1882.

153. Nazhat S.N., Joseph R., Wang M., Smith R., Tanner K.E., Bonfield W., Dynamic mechanical characterisation of hydroxyapatite reinforced polyethylene: effect of particle size. *J. Mater. Sci. Mater. Med.*, (2000), 11, 621–628.

154. Guild F.J., Bonfield W., Predictive modelling of the mechanical properties and failure processes of hydroxyapatite-polyethylene (HAPEX™) composite. *J. Mater. Sci. Mater. Med.*, (1998), 9, 497–502.

155. Wang M., Ladizesky N.H., Tanner K.E., Ward I.M., Bonfield W., Hydrostatically extruded HAPEX™. *J. Mater. Sci.*, (2000), 35, 1023–1030.

156. That P.T., Tanner K.E., Bonfield W., Fatigue characterization of a hydroxyapatite-reinforced polyethylene composite. I. Uniaxial fatigue. *J. Biomed. Mater. Res.*, (2000), 51, 453–460.

157. That P.T., Tanner K.E., Bonfield W., Fatigue characterization of a hydroxyapatite-reinforced polyethylene composite. II. Biaxial fatigue. *J. Biomed. Mater. Res.*, (2000), 51, 461–468.

158. Bonner M., Saunders L.S., Ward I.M., Davies G.W., Wang M., Tanner K.E., Bonfield W., Anisotropic mechanical properties of oriented HAPEX™. *J. Mater. Sci.*, (2002), 37, 325–334.

159. di Silvio L., Dalby M.J., Bonfield W., Osteoblast behaviour on HA/PE composite surfaces with different HA volumes. *Biomaterials*, (2002), 23, 101–107.

160. Dalby M.J., Kayser M.V., Bonfield W., di Silvio L., Initial attachment of osteoblasts to an optimised HAPEX™ topography. *Biomaterials*, (2002), 23, 681–690.

161. Zhang Y., Tanner K.E., Gurav N., di Silvio L., *In vitro* osteoblastic response to 30 vol% hydroxyapatite-polyethylene composite. *J. Biomed. Mater. Res. A*, (2007), 81A, 409–417.

162. Rea S.M., Brooks R.A., Schneider A., Best S.M., Bonfield W. Osteoblast-like cell response to bioactive composites-surface-topography and composition effects. *J. Biomed. Mater. Res. B Appl. Biomater.*, (2004), 70B, 250–261.

163. Salernitano E., Migliaresi C., Composite materials for biomedical applications: a review. *J. Appl. Biomater. Biomech.*, (2003), 1, 3–18.

164. Pandey A., Jan E., Aswath P.B., Physical and mechanical behavior of hot rolled HDPE/HA composites. *J. Mater. Sci.*, (2006), 41, 3369–3376.

165. Bonner M., Ward I.M., McGregor W., Tanner K.E., Bonfield W. Hydroxyapatite/polypropylene composite: a novel bone substitute material. *J. Mater. Sci. Lett.*, (2001), 20, 2049–2052.

166. Suppakarn N., Sanmaung S., Ruksakulpiwa Y., Sutapun W., Effect of surface modification on properties of natural hydroxyapatite/polypropylene composites. *Key Eng. Mater.*, (2008), 361-363, 511–514.

167. Younesi M., Bahrololoom M.E., Formulating the effects of applied temperature and pressure of hot pressing process on the mechanical properties of polypropylene-hydroxyapatite bio-composites by response surface methodology. *Mater. Des.*, (2010), 31, 4621–4630.

168. Younesi M., Bahrololoom M.E., Effect of polypropylene molecular weight, hydroxyapatite particle size, and Ringer's solution on creep and impact behavior of polypropylene-surface treated hydroxyapatite biocomposites. *J. Compos. Mater.*, (2011), 45, 513–523.

169. Sousa R.A., Reis R.L., Cunha A.M., Bevis M.J., Processing and properties of bone-analogue biodegradable and bioinert polymeric composites. *Compos. Sci. Technol.*, (2003), 63, 389–402.

170. Wang M., Deb S., Bonfield W., Chemically coupled hydroxyapatite-polyethylene composites: processing and characterisation. *Mater. Lett.*, (2000), 44, 119–124.

171. Wang M., Bonfield W., Chemically coupled hydroxyapatite-polyethylene composites: structure and properties. *Biomaterials*, (2001), 22, 1311–1320.

172. Homaeigohar S.S., Shokrgozar M.A., Khavandi A., Sadi A.Y., *In vitro* biological evaluation of β-TCP/HDPE – a novel orthopedic composite: a survey using human osteoblast and fibroblast bone cells. *J. Biomed. Mater. Res. A*, (2008), 84A, 491–499.

173. Sadi A.Y., Homaeigohar S.Sh., Khavandi A.R., Javadpour J., The effect of partially stabilized zirconia on the mechanical properties of the hydroxyapatite-polyethylene composites. *J. Mater. Sci. Mater. Med.*, (2004), 15, 853–858.

174. Nath S., Bodhak S., Basu B. HDPE-Al$_2$O$_3$-HAp composites for biomedical applications: processing and characterizations. *J. Biomed. Mater. Res. B Appl. Biomater.*, (2009), 88B, 1–11.

175. Downes R.N., Vardy S., Tanner K.E., Bonfield W. Hydroxyapatite-polyethylene composite in orbital surgery. *Bioceramics*, (1991), 4, 239–246.

176. Dornhoffer H.L., Hearing results with the Dornhoffer ossicular replacement prostheses. *Laryngoscope*, (1998), 108, 531–536.

177. Swain R.E., Wang M., Beale B., Bonfield W. HAPEX™ for otologic applications. *Biomed. Eng. Appl. Basis Commun.*, (1999), 11, 315–320.

178. Yi Z., Li Y., Jidong L., Xiang Z., Hongbing L., Yuanyuan W., Weihu Y., Novel bio-composite of hydroxyapatite reinforced polyamide and polyethylene: composition and properties. *Mater. Sci. Eng. A*, (2007), 452–453, 512–517.

179. Unwin A.P., Ward I., M., Ukleja P., Weng J., The role of pressure annealing in improving the stiffness of polyethylene/hydroxyapatite composites. *J. Mater. Sci.*, (2001), 36, 3165–3177.

180. Fang L.M., Leng Y., Gao P., Processing and mechanical properties of HA/UHMWPE nanocomposites. *Biomaterials*, (2006), 27, 3701–3707.

181. Fang L.M., Gao P., Leng Y., High strength and bioactive hydroxyapatite nano-particles reinforced ultrahigh molecular weight polyethylene. *Composites B*, (2007), 38, 345–351.

182. Fang L.M., Leng Y., Gao P., Processing of hydroxyapatite reinforced ultrahigh molecular weight polyethylene for biomedical applications. *Biomaterials*, (2005), 26, 3471–3478.

183. Selvin T.P., Seno J., Murukan B., Santhosh A.A., Sabu T., Weimin Y., Sri B. Poly(ethylene-*co*-vinyl acetate)/calcium phosphate nanocomposites: thermo mechanical and gas permeability measurements. *Polym. Comp.*, (2010), 31, 1011–1019.

184. Reis R.L., Cunha A.M., Oliveira M.J., Campos A.R., Bevis M.J., Relationship between processing and mechanical properties of injection molded high molecular mass polyethylene + hydroxyapatite composites. *Mater. Res. Inn.*, (2001), 4, 263–272.

185. Sousa R.A., Reis R.L., Cunha A.M., Bevis M.J., Structure development and interfacial interactions in high-density polyethylene/hydroxyapatite (HDPE/HA) composites molded with preferred orientation. *J. Appl. Polym. Sci.*, (2002), 86, 2873–2886.

186. Mirsalehi S.A., Khavandi A., Mirdamadi S., Naimi-Jamal M.R., Kalantari S.M., Nanomechanical and tribological behavior of hydroxyapatite reinforced ultrahigh molecular weight polyethylene nanocomposites for biomedical applications. *J. Appl. Polym. Sci.*, (2015), 132, 42052.

187. Donners J.J.J.M., Nolte R.J.M., Sommerdijk N.A.J.M. Dendrimer-based hydroxyapatite composites with remarkable materials properties. *Adv. Mater.*, (2003), 15, 313–316.

188. Schneider O.D., Stepuk A., Mohn D., Luechinger N.A., Feldman K., Stark W.J. Light-curable polymer/calcium phosphate nanocomposite glue for bone defect treatment. *Acta Biomater.*, (2010), 6, 2704–2710.

189. Ignjatovic N.L., Plavsic M., Miljkovic M.S., Zivkovic L.M., Uskokovic D.P., Microstructural characteristics of calcium hydroxyapatite/poly-L-lactide based composites. *J. Microsc.*, (1999), 196, 243–248.

190. Skrtic D., Antonucci J.M., Eanes E.D., Amorphous calcium phosphate-based bioactive polymeric composites for mineralized tissue regeneration. *J. Res. Natl. Inst. Stand. Technol.*, (2003), 108, 167–182.

191. Rizzi S.C., Heath D.J., Coombes A.G., A., Bock N., Textor M., Downes S., Biodegradable polymer/hydroxyapatite composites: surface analysis and initial attachment of human osteoblasts. *J. Biomed. Mater. Res.*, (2001), 55, 475–486.

192. Navarro M., Planell J.A., Bioactive composites based on calcium phosphates for bone regeneration. *Key Eng. Mater.*, (2010), 441, 203–233.

193. Zhang R.Y., Ma P.X., Porous poly(L-lactic acid)/apatite composites created by biomimetic process. *J. Biomed. Mater. Res.*, (1999), 45, 285–293.

194. Liu Q., de Wijn J.R., van Blitterswijk C.A., Composite biomaterials with chemical bonding between hydroxyapatite filler particles and PEG/PBT copolymer matrix. *J. Biomed. Mater. Res.*, (1998), 40, 490–497.

195. Cerrai P., Guerra G.D., Tricoli M., Krajewski A., Ravaglioli A., Martinetti R., Dolcini L., Fini M., Scarano A., Piattelli A., Periodontal membranes from composites of hydroxyapatite and bioresorbable block copolymers. *J. Mater. Sci. Mater. Med.*, (1999), 10, 677–682.

196. Roeder R.K., Sproul M.M., Turner C.H., Hydroxyapatite whiskers provide improved mechanical properties in reinforced polymer composites. *J. Biomed. Mater. Res. A*, (2003), 67A, 801–812.

197. Wagoner Johnson A.J., Herschler B.A., A review of the mechanical behavior of CaP and CaP/polymer composites for applications in bone replacement and repair. *Acta Biomater.*, (2011), 7, 16–30.

198. Hutmacher D.W., Scaffolds in tissue engineering bone and cartilage. *Biomaterials*, (2000), 21, 2529–2543.

199. Mathieu L.M., Bourban P.E., Manson J.A.E., Processing of homogeneous ceramic/polymer blends for bioresorbable composites. *Compos. Sci. Technol.*, (2006), 66, 1606–1614.

200. Redepenning J., Venkataraman G., Chen J., Stafford N., Electrochemical preparation of chitosan/hydroxyapatite composite coatings on titanium substrates. *J. Biomed. Mater. Res. A*, (2003), 66A, 411–416.

201. Rhee S.H., Tanaka J., Synthesis of a hydroxyapatite/collagen/chondroitin sulfate nanocomposite by a novel precipitation method. *J. Am. Ceram. Soc.*, (2001), 84, 459–461.

202. Pezzotti G., Asmus S.M.F., Fracture behavior of hydroxyapatite/polymer interpenetrating network composites prepared by *in situ* polymerization process. *Mater. Sci. Eng. A*, (2001), 316, 231–237.

203. Weickmann H., Gurr M., Meincke O., Thomann R., Mülhaupt R., A versatile solvent-free "one-pot" route to polymer nanocomposites and the *in situ* formation of calcium phosphate/layered silicate hybrid nanoparticles. *Adv. Funct. Mater.*, (2010), 20, 1778–1786.

204. Aryal S., Bhattarai S.R., Bahadur K.C.R., Khil M.S., Lee D.R., Kim H.Y., Carbon nanotubes assisted biomimetic synthesis of hydroxyapatite from simulated body fluid. *Mater. Sci. Eng. A*, (2006), 426, 202–207.

205. Kealley C., Ben-Nissan B., van Riessen A., Elcombe M., Development of carbon nanotube reinforced hydroxyapatite bioceramics. *Key Eng. Mater.*, (2006), 309–311, 597–600.

206. Kealley C., Elcombe M., van Riessen A., Ben-Nissan B., Development of carbon nanotube reinforced hydroxyapatite bioceramics. *Physica B*, (2006), 385–386, 496–498.

207. Aryal S., Bahadur K.C.R., Dharmaraj N., Kim K.W., Kim H.Y., Synthesis and characterization of hydroxyapatite using carbon nanotubes as a nano-matrix. *Scripta Mater.*, (2006), 54, 131–135.

208. Rautaray D., Mandal S., Sastry M., Synthesis of hydroxyapatite crystals using amino acid-capped gold nanoparticles as a scaffold. *Langmuir*, (2005), 21, 5185–5191.

209. Wang X.J., Li Y., Wei J., de Groot K., Development of biomimetic nano-hydroxyapatite/poly(hexamethylene adipamide) composites. *Biomaterials*, (2002), 23, 4787–4791.

210. Wei J., Li Y., Tissue engineering scaffold material of nano-apatite crystals and polyamide composite. *Eur. Polym. J.*, (2004), 40, 509–515.

211. Memoto R., Nakamura S., Isobe T., Senna M., Direct synthesis of hydroxyapatite-silk fibroin nano-composite sol via a mechano-chemical route. *J. Sol Gel Sci. Technol.*, (2001), 21, 7–12.

212. Yoshida A., Miyazaki T., Ashizuka M., Ishida E., Bioactivity and mechanical properties of cellulose/carbonate hydroxyapatite composites prepared *in situ* through mechanochemical reaction. *J. Biomater. Appl.*, (2006), 21, 179–194.

213. Fujiwara M., Shiokawa K., Morigaki K., Tatsu Y., Nakahara Y., Calcium phosphate composite materials including inorganic powders, BSA or duplex DNA prepared by W/O/W interfacial reaction method. *Mater. Sci. Eng. C*, (2008), 28, 280–288.

214. Nagata F., Miyajima T., Yokogawa Y., A method to fabricate hydroxyapatite/poly(lactic acid) microspheres intended for biomedical application. *J. Eur. Ceram. Soc.*, (2006), 26, 533–535.

215. Russias J., Saiz E., Nalla R.K., Tomsia A.P., Microspheres as building blocks for hydroxyapatite/polylactide biodegradable composites. *J. Mater. Sci.*, (2006), 41, 5127–5133.

216. Khan Y.M., Cushnie E.K., Kelleher J.K., Laurencin C.T., *In situ* synthesized ceramic-polymer composites for bone tissue engineering: bioactivity and degradation studies. *J. Mater. Sci.*, (2007), 42, 4183–4190.

217. Liu X., Okada M., Maeda H., Fujii S., Furuzono T. Hydroxyapatite/biodegradable poly(L-lactide-*co*-ε-caprolactone) composite microparticles as injectable scaffolds by a Pickering emulsion route. *Acta Biomater.*, (2011), 7, 821–828.

218. Hu Y., Zou S., Chen W., Tong Z., Wang C., Mineralization and drug release of hydroxyapatite/poly(L-lactic acid) nanocomposite scaffolds prepared by Pickering emulsion templating. *Colloid Surface B*, (2014), 122, 559–565.

219. Kim H.W., Knowles J.C., Kim H.E., Hydroxyapatite and gelatin composite foams processed via novel freeze-drying and crosslinking for use as temporary hard tissue scaffolds. *J. Biomed. Mater. Res. A*, (2005), 72A, 136–145.

220. Mohandes F., Salavati-Niasari M. Freeze-drying synthesis, characterization and *in vitro* bioactivity of chitosan/graphene oxide/hydroxyapatite nanocomposite. *RSC Adv.*, (2014), 4, 25993–26001.

221. Sinha A., Das G., Sharma B.K., Roy R.P., Pramanick A.K., Nayar S. Poly(vinyl alcohol)-hydroxyapatite biomimetic scaffold for tissue regeneration. *Mater. Sci. Eng. C*, (2007), 27, 70–74.

222. Sugawara A., Yamane S., Akiyoshi K. Nanogel-templated mineralization: polymer-calcium phosphate hybrid nanomaterials. *Macromol. Rapid Commun.*, (2006), 27, 441–446.
223. Kickelbick G., Concepts for the incorporation of inorganic building blocks into organic polymers on a nanoscale. *Prog. Polym. Sci.*, (2003), 28, 83–114.
224. Liu Q., de Wijn J.R., van Blitterswijk C.A. Nanoapatite/polymer composites: mechanical and physicochemical characteristics. *Biomaterials*, (1997), 18, 1263–1270.
225. Uskokovic P.S., Tang C.Y., Tsui C.P., Ignjatovic N., Uskokovic D.P., Micromechanical properties of a hydroxyapatite/poly-L-lactide biocomposite using nanoindentation and modulus mapping. *J. Eur. Ceram. Soc.*, (2007), 27, 1559–1564.
226. Todo M., Kagawa T., Improvement of fracture energy of HA/PLLA biocomposite material due to press processing. *J. Mater. Sci.*, (2008), 43, 799–801.
227. Woo K.M., Seo J., Zhang R.Y., Ma P.X., Suppression of apoptosis by enhanced protein adsorption on polymer/hydroxyapatite composite scaffolds. *Biomaterials*, (2007), 28, 2622–2630.
228. Baji A., Wong S.C., Srivatsan T.S., Njus G.O., Mathur G., Processing methodologies for polycaprolactone-hydroxyapatite composites: a review. *Mater. Manuf. Process.*, (2006), 21, 211–218.
229. Guan L., Davies J.E., Preparation and characterization of a highly macroporous biodegradable composite tissue engineering scaffold. *J. Biomed. Mater. Res. A*, (2004), 71A, 480–487.
230. Sun F., Zhou H., Lee J., Various preparation methods of highly porous hydroxyapatite/polymer nanoscale biocomposites for bone regeneration. *Acta Biomater.*, (2011), 7, 3813–3828.
231. Kumar A., Negi Y.S., Choudhary V., Bhardwaj N.K., Microstructural and mechanical properties of porous biocomposite scaffolds based on polyvinyl alcohol, nano-hydroxyapatite and cellulose nanocrystals. *Cellulose*, (2015), 21, 3409–3426.
232. Teng X.R., Ren J., Gu S.Y., Preparation and characterization of porous PDLLA/HA composite foams by supercritical carbon dioxide technology. *J. Biomed. Mater. Res. B Appl. Biomater.*, (2007), 81B, 185–193.
233. Ren J., Zhao P., Ren T., Gu S., Pan K., Poly (D,L-lactide)/nano-hydroxyapatite composite scaffolds for bone tissue engineering and biocompatibility evaluation. *J. Mater. Sci. Mater. Med.*, (2008), 19, 1075–1082.
234. Wang M., Yue C.Y., Chua B., Production and evaluation of hydroxyapatite reinforced polysulfone for tissue replacement. *J. Mater. Sci. Mater. Med.*, (2001), 12, 821–826.
235. Chlopek J., Rosol P., Morawska-Chochol A., Durability of polymer-ceramics composite implants determined in creep tests. *Compos. Sci. Technol.*, (2006), 66, 1615–1622.

236. Robinson P., Wilson C., Mecholsky J., Processing and mechanical properties of hydroxyapatite-polysulfone laminated composites. *J. Eur. Ceram. Soc.*, (2014), 34, 1387–1396.

237. Xu F., Li Y., Yao X., Liao H., Zhang L., Preparation and *in vivo* investigation of artificial cornea made of nano-hydroxyapatite/poly (vinyl alcohol) hydrogel composite. *J. Mater. Sci. Mater. Med.*, (2007), 18, 635–640.

238. Xu F., Li Y., Deng Y., Xiong G., Porous nano-hydroxyapatite/poly(vinyl alcohol) composite hydrogel as artificial cornea fringe: characterization and evaluation *in vitro*. *J. Biomater. Sci. Polym. Edn.*, (2008), 19, 431–439.

239. Nayar S., Pramanick A.K., Sharma B.K., Das G., Kumar B.R., Sinha A., Biomimetically synthesized polymer-hydroxyapatite sheet like nanocomposite. *J. Mater. Sci. Mater. Med.*, (2008), 19, 301–304.

240. Poursamar S.A., Orang F., Bonakdar S., Savar M.K., Preparation and characterisation of poly vinyl alcohol/hydroxyapatite nanocomposite via *in situ* synthesis: a potential material as bone tissue engineering scaffolds. *Int. J. Nanomanuf.*, (2010), 5, 330–334.

241. Guha A., Nayar S., Thatoi H.N., Microwave irradiation enhances kinetics of the biomimetic process of hydroxyapatite nanocomposites. *Bioinspir. Biomim.*, (2010) 5, 024001 (5 pages).

242. Timofejeva A., Loca D. Hydroxyapatite/polyvinyl alcohol composite hydrogels for bone and cartilage tissue engineering. *Key Eng. Mater.*, (2018), 762, 54–58.

243. Pramanik N., Biswas S.K., Pramanik P., Synthesis and characterization of hydroxyapatite/poly(vinyl alcohol phosphate) nanocomposite biomaterials. *Int. J. Appl. Ceram. Technol.*, (2008), 5, 20–28.

244. Bigi A., Boanini E., Gazzano M., Rubini K., Structural and morphological modifications of hydroxyapatite-polyaspartate composite crystals induced by heat treatment. *Cryst. Res. Technol.*, (2005), 40, 1094–1098.

245. Bertoni E., Bigi A., Falini G., Panzavolta S., Roveri N., Hydroxyapatite polyacrylic acid nanocrystals. *J. Mater. Chem.*, (1999), 9, 779–782.

246. Qiu H.J., Yang J., Kodali P., Koh J., Ameer G.A., A citric acid-based hydroxyapatite composite for orthopedic implants. *Biomaterials*, (2006), 27, 5845–5854.

247. Greish Y.E., Brown P.W., Chemically formed HAp-Ca poly(vinyl phosphonate) composites. *Biomaterials*, (2001), 22, 807–816.

248. Greish Y.E., Brown P.W., Preparation and characterization of calcium phosphate-poly(vinyl phosphonic acid) composites. *J. Mater. Sci. Mater. Med.*, (2001), 12, 407–411.

249. Greish Y.E., Brown P.W., Formation and properties of hydroxyapatite-calcium poly(vinyl phosphonate) composites. *J. Am. Ceram. Soc.*, (2002), 85, 1738–1744.

250. Sailaja G.S., Velayudhan S., Sunny M.C., Sreenivasan K., Varma H.K., Ramesh P., Hydroxyapatite filled chitosan-polyacrylic acid polyelectrolyte complexes. *J. Mater. Sci.*, (2003), 38, 3653–3662.

251. Piticescu R.M., Chitanu G.C., Albulescu M., Giurginca M., Popescu M.L., Łojkowski W., Hybrid HAp-maleic anhydride copolymer nanocomposites obtained by in-situ functionalisation. *Solid State Phenom.*, (2005), 106, 47–56.

252. Song J., Saiz E., Bertozzi C.R., A new approach to mineralization of biocompatible hydrogel scaffolds: an efficient process toward 3-dimensional bonelike composites. *J. Am. Chem. Soc.*, (2003), 125, 1236–1243.

253. Kutikov A.B., Song J., An amphiphilic degradable polymer/hydroxyapatite composite with enhanced handling characteristics promotes osteogenic gene expression in bone marrow stromal cells. *Acta Biomater.*, (2013), 9, 8354–8364.

254. Wu S., Wang J., Zou L., Jin L., Wang Z., Li Y., A three-dimensional hydroxyapatite/polyacrylonitrile composite scaffold designed for bone tissue engineering. *RSC Adv.*, (2018), 8, 1730–1736.

255. Borkowski L., Lübek T., Jojczuk M., Nogalski A., Belcarz A., Hajnos M., Ginalska G., Behavior of new hydroxyapatite/glucan composite in human serum. *J. Biomed. Mater. Res. B Appl. Biomater.*, (2018), doi: 10.1002/jbm.b.34082.

256. Abu Bakar M.S., Cheng M.H.W., Tang S.M., Yu S.C., Liao K., Tan C.T., Khor K.A., Cheang P., Tensile properties, tension–tension fatigue and biological response of polyetheretherketone–hydroxyapatite composites for load-bearing orthopedic implants. *Biomaterials*, (2003), 24, 2245–2250.

257. Abu Bakar M.S., Cheang P., Khor K.A., Mechanical properties of injection molded hydroxyapatite-polyetheretherketone biocomposites. *Compos. Sci. Technol.*, (2003), 63, 421–425.

258. Abu Bakar M.S., Cheang P., Khor K.A., Tensile properties and microstructural analysis of spheroidized hydroxyapatite-poly (etheretherketone) biocomposites. *Mater. Sci. Eng. A*, (2003), 345, 55–63.

259. Fan J.P., Tsui C.P., Tang C.Y., Modeling of the mechanical behavior of HA/PEEK biocomposite under quasi-static tensile load. *Mater. Sci. Eng. A*, (2004), 382, 341–350.

260. Wang L., Weng L., Song S., Sun Q., Mechanical properties and microstructure of polyetheretherketone-hydroxyapatite nanocomposite materials. *Mater. Lett.*, (2010), 64, 2201–2204.

261. Li K., Yeung C.Y., Yeung K.W.K., Tjong S.C., Sintered hydroxyapatite/polyetheretherketone nanocomposites: mechanical behavior and biocompatibility. *Adv. Eng. Mater.*, (2012), 14, B155–B165.

262. Wang L., He S., Wu X., Liang S., Mu Z., Wei J., Deng F., Deng Y., Wei S. Polyetheretherketone/nano-fluorohydroxyapatite composite with antimicrobial activity and osseointegration properties. *Biomaterials*, (2014), 35, 6758–6775.

263. Gong X.H., Tang C.Y., Hu H.C., Zhou X.P., Improved mechanical properties of HIPS/hydroxyapatite composites by surface modification of hydroxyapatite via *in situ* polymerization of styrene. *J. Mater. Sci. Mater. Med.*, (2004), 15, 1141–1146.

264. Fu G., Xia Z., Jiang J., Jing B., Zhang X., Fabrication and characterization of nanocomposites with high-impact polystyrene and hydroxyapatite with well-defined polystyrene via ATRP. *J. Reinf. Plast. Comp.*, (2011), 30, 1445–1453.

265. Petricca S.E., Marra K.G., Kumta P.N., Chemical synthesis of poly(lactic-*co*-glycolic acid)/hydroxyapatite composites for orthopaedic applications. *Acta Biomater.*, (2006), 2, 277–286.

266. Kim S.S., Ahn K.M., Park M.S., Lee J.H., Choi C.Y., Kim B.S. A poly(lactide-*co*-glycolide)/hydroxyapatite composite scaffold with enhanced osteoconductivity. *J. Biomed. Mater. Res. A*, (2007), 80A, 206–215.

267. Oliveira J., Miyazaki T., Lopes M., Ohtsuki C., Santos J., Bonelike®/PLGA hybrid materials for bone regeneration: preparation route and physicochemical characterization. *J. Mater. Sci. Mater. Med.*, (2005), 16, 253–259.

268. Aboudzadeh N., Imani M., Shokrgozar M.A., Khavandi A., Javadpour J., Shafieyan Y., Farokhi M., Fabrication and characterization of poly(D,L-lactide-*co*-glycolide)/ hydroxyapatite nanocomposite scaffolds for bone tissue regeneration. *J. Biomed. Mater. Res. A*, (2010), 94A, 137–145.

269. Zhou H., Lawrence J.G., Bhaduri S.B., Fabrication aspects of PLA-CaP/PLGA-CaP composites for orthopedic applications: a review. *Acta Biomater.*, (2012), 8, 1999–2016.

270. Hoekstra J.W.M., Ma J., Plachokova A.S., Bronkhorst E.M., Bohner M., Pan J., Meijer G.J., Jansen J.A., van den Beucken J.J.J.P., The *in vivo* performance of CaP/PLGA composites with varied PLGA microsphere sizes and inorganic compositions. *Acta Biomater.*, (2013), 9, 7518–7526.

271. Leung L.H., Naguib H.E., Characterizing the viscoelastic behaviour of poly(lactide-*co*-glycolide acid)–hydroxyapatite foams. *J. Cell. Plast.*, (2013), 49, 497–505.

272. Takeoka Y., Hayashi M., Sugiyama N., Yoshizawa-Fujita M., Aizawa M., Rikukawa M., *In situ* preparation of poly(l-lactic acid-*co*-glycolic acid)/hydroxyapatite composites as artificial bone materials. *Polym. J.*, (2015), 47, 164–170.

273. Fisher P.D., Venugopal G., Milbrandt T.A., Hilt J.Z., Puleo D.A., Hydroxyapatite-reinforced *in situ* forming PLGA systems for intraosseous injection. *J. Biomed. Mater. Res. A*, (2015), 103A, 2365–2373.

274. Athanasiou K.A., Schmitz J.P., Agrawal C.M., The effects of porosity on *in vitro* degradation of polylactic acid- polyglycolic acid implants used in repair of articular cartilage. *Tissue Eng.*, (1998), 4, 53–63.

275. Verheyen C.C.P.M., Klein C.P.A.T., de Blieck-Hogervorst J.M.A., Wolke J.G.C., de Wijin J.R., van Blitterswijk C.A., de Groot K., Evaluation of hydroxylapatite poly(L-lactide) composites: physico-chemical properties. *J. Mater. Sci. Mater. Med.*, (1993), 4, 58–65.

276. Agrawal C.M., Athanasiou K.A., Technique to control pH in vicinity of biodegrading PLA-PGA implants. *J. Biomed. Mater. Res. Appl. Biomater.*, (1997), 38, 105–114.

277. Li H., Chang J. pH-compensation effect of bioactive inorganic fillers on the degradation of PLGA. *Compos. Sci. Technol.*, (2005), 65, 2226–2232.

278. Peter S.J., Miller S.T., Zhu G., Yasko A.W., Mikos A.G., *In vivo* degradation of a poly(propylene fumarate)/β-tricalcium phosphate injectable composite scaffold. *J. Biomed. Mater. Res.*, (1998), 41, 1–7.

279. Ara M., Watanabe M., Imai Y., Effect of blending calcium compounds on hydrolitic degradation of poly(D,L-lactic acid-co-glycolic acid). *Biomaterials*, (2002), 23, 2479–2483.

280. Linhart W., Peters F., Lehmann W., Schwarz K., Schilling A., Amling M., Rueger J.M., Epple M., Biologically and chemically optimized composites of carbonated apatite and polyglycolide as bone substitution materials. *J. Biomed. Mater. Res.*, (2001), 54, 162–171.

281. Schiller C., Epple M., Carbonated apatites can be used as pH-stabilizing filler for biodegradable polyesters. *Biomaterials*, (2003), 24, 2037–2043.

282. Schiller C., Rasche C., Wehmöller M., Beckmann F., Eufinger H., Epple M., Weihe S., Geometrically structured implants for cranial reconstruction made of biodegradable polyesters and calcium phosphate/calcium carbonate. *Biomaterials*, (2004), 25, 1239–1247.

283. Shikinami Y., Okuno M., Bioresorbable devices made of forged composites of hydroxyapatite (HA) particles and poly L-lactide (PLLA). Part II: practical properties of miniscrews and miniplates. *Biomaterials*, (2001), 22, 3197–3211.

284. Russias J., Saiz E., Nalla R.K., Gryn K., Ritchie R.O., Tomsia A.P., Fabrication and mechanical properties of PLA/HA composites: a study of *in vitro* degradation. *Mater. Sci. Eng. C*, (2006), 26, 1289–1295.

285. Akagi H., Iwata M., Ichinohe T., Amimoto H., Hayashi Y., Kannno N., Ochi H., Fujita Y., Harada Y., Tagawa M., Hara Y. Hydroxyapatite/poly-L-lactide acid screws have better biocompatibility and femoral burr hole closure than does poly-L-lactide acid alone. *J. Biomater. Appl.*, (2014), 28, 954–962.

286. Kim H.W., Lee H.H., Knowles J.C., Electrospinning biomedical nanocomposite fibers of hydroxyapaite/poly(lactic acid) for bone regeneration. *J. Biomed. Mater. Res. A*, (2006), 79A, 643–649.

287. Gross K.A., Rodríguez-Lorenzo L.M., Biodegradable composite scaffolds with an interconnected spherical network for bone tissue engineering. *Biomaterials*, (2004), 25, 4955–4962.

288. Zhang H., Chen Z., Fabrication and characterization of electrospun PLGA/MWNTs/ hydroxyapatite biocomposite scaffolds for bone tissue engineering. *J. Bioact. Compat. Polym.*, (2010), 25, 241–259.

289. Durucan C., Brown P.W., Low temperature formation of calcium-deficient hydroxyapatite-PLA/PLGA composites. *J. Biomed. Mater. Res.*, (2000), 51, 717–725.

290. Durucan C., Brown P.W., Calcium-deficient hydroxyapatite-PLGA composites: mechanical and microstructural investigation. *J. Biomed. Mater. Res.*, (2000), 51, 726–734.

291. Durucan C., Brown P.W., Biodegradable hydroxyapatite-polymer composites. *Adv. Eng. Mater.*, (2001), 3, 227–231.

292. Nazhat S.N., Kellomäki M., Törmälä, P., Tanner K.E., Bonfield W., Dynamic mechanical characterization of biodegradable composites of hydroxyapatite and polylactides. *J. Biomed. Mater. Res.*, (2001), 58, 335–343.

293. Ignjatovic N., Suljovrujic E., Biudinski-Simendic J., Krakovsky I., Uskokovic D., Evaluation of hot-presses hydroxyapatite/poly-L-lactide composite biomaterial characteristics. *J. Biomed. Mater. Res. B Appl. Biomater.*, (2004), 71B, 284–294.

294. Wang X., Lou T., Yang J., Yang Z., He K., Preparation of PLLA/ HAP/β-TCP composite scaffold for bone tissue engineering. *Appl. Mech. Mater.*, (2014), 513–517, 143–146.

295. Hasegawa S., Tamura J., Neo M., Goto K., Shikinami Y., Saito M., Kita M., Nakamura T., *In vivo* evaluation of a porous hydroxyapatite/poly-D,L-lactide composite for use as a bone substitute. *J. Biomed. Mater. Res. A*, (2005), 75A, 567–579.

296. Hasegawa S., Neo M., Tamura J., Fujibayashi S., Takemoto M., Shikinami Y., Okazaki K., Nakamura T., *In vivo* evaluation of a porous hydroxyapatite/poly-D,L-lactide composite for bone tissue engineering. *J. Biomed. Mater. Res. A*, (2007), 81A, 930–938.

297. Kim S.S., Park M.S., Jeon Q., Choi C.Y., Kim B.S. Poly(lactide-*co*-glycolide)/hydroxyapatite composite scaffolds for bone tissue engineering. *Biomaterials*, (2006), 27, 1399–1409.

298. Mao D., Li Q., Bai N., Dong H., Li D., Porous stable poly(lactic acid)/ ethyl cellulose/hydroxyapatite composite scaffolds prepared by a combined method for bone regeneration. *Carbohyd. Polym.*, (2018), 180, 104–111.

299. Reis R.L., Cunha A.M., New degradable load-bearing biomaterials composed of reinforced starch based blends. *J. Appl. Med. Polym.*, (2000), 4, 1–5.

300. Sousa R.A., Mano J.F., Reis R.L., Cunha A.M., Bevis M.J., Mechanical performance of starch based bioactive composites moulded with preferred orientation for potential medical applications. *Polym. Eng. Sci.*, (2002), 42, 1032–1045.

301. Marques A.P., Reis R.L., Hydroxyapatite reinforcement of different starch-based polymers affects osteoblast-like cells adhesion/spreading and proliferation. *Mater. Sci. Eng. C*, (2005), 25, 215–229.
302. Reis R.L., Cunha A.M., Allan P.S., Bevis M.J., Structure development and control of injection-molded hydroxylapatite-reinforced starch/EVOH composites. *Adv. Polym. Tech.*, (1997), 16, 263–277.
303. Vaz C.M., Reis R.L., Cunha A.M., Use of coupling agents to enhance the interfacial interactions in starch-EVOH/hydroxylapatite composites. *Biomaterials*, (2002), 23, 629–635.
304. Leonor I.B., Ito A., Onuma K., Kanzaki N., Reis R.L., *In vitro* bioactivity of starch thermoplastic/hydroxyapatite composite biomaterials: an *in situ* study using atomic force microscopy. *Biomaterials*, (2003), 24, 579–585.
305. Vaz C.M., Reis R.L., Cunha A.M., Degradation model of starch-EVOH+HA composites. *Mater. Res. Innov.*, (2001), 4, 375–380.
306. Chen L.J., Wang M., Production and evaluation of biodegradable composites based on PHB-PHV copolymer. *Biomaterials*, (2002), 23, 2631–2639.
307. Ni J., Wang M., *In vitro* evaluation of hydroxyapatite reinforced polyhydroxybutyrate composite. *Mater. Sci. Eng. C*, (2002), 20, 101–109.
308. Carlo E.C., Borges A.P.B., Del Carlo R.J., Martinez M.M.M., Oliveira P.M., Morato G.O., Eleotério R.B., Reis M.S., Comparison of *in vivo* properties of hydroxyapatite-polyhydroxybutyrate composites assessed for bone substitution. *J. Craniofac. Surg.*, (2009), 20, 853–859.
309. Reis E.C.C., Borges A.P.B., Fonseca C.C., Martinez M.M.M., Eleotério R.B., Morato G.O., Oliveira P.M. Biocompatibility, osteointegration, osteoconduction, and biodegradation of a hydroxyapatite-polyhydroxybutyrate composite. *Braz. Arch. Biol. Technol.*, (2010), 53, 817–826.
310. Sadat-Shojai M., Khorasani M.T., Jamshidi A., Irani S. Nano-hydroxyapatite reinforced polyhydroxybutyrate composites: a comprehensive study on the structural and *in vitro* biological properties. *Mater. Sci. Eng. C*, (2013), 33, 2776–2787.
311. Chen D.Z., Tang C.Y., Chan K.C., Tsui C.P., Yu P.H.F., Leung M.C.P., Uskokovic P.S., Dynamic mechanical properties and *in vitro* bioactivity of PHBHV/HA nanocomposite. *Compos. Sci. Technol.*, (2007), 67, 1617–1626.
312. Rai B., Noohom W., Kithva P.H., Grøndahl L., Trau M., Bionanohydroxyapatite/poly(3-hydroxybutyrate-*co*-3-hydroxyvalerate) composites with improved particle dispersion and superior mechanical properties. *Chem. Mater.*, (2008), 20, 2802–2808.
313. Wang Y.W., Wu Q., Chen J., Chen G.Q., Evaluation of three-dimensional scaffolds made of blends of hydroxyapatite and poly(3-hydroxybutyrate-*co*-3-hydroxyhexanoate) for bone reconstruction. *Biomaterials*, (2005), 26, 899–904.

314. Linhart W., Lehmann W., Siedler M., Peters F., Schilling A.F., Schwarz K., Amling M., Rueger J.M., Epple M., Composites of amorphous calcium phosphate and poly(hydroxybutyrate) and poly(hydroxybutyrate-*co*-hydroxyvalerate) for bone substitution: assessment of the biocompatibility. *J. Mater. Sci.*, (2006), 41, 4806–4813.

315. Azevedo M., Reis R.L., Claase M., Grijpma D., Feijen J., Development and properties of polycaprolactone/hydroxyapatite composite biomaterials. *J. Mater. Sci. Mater. Med.*, (2003), 14, 103–107.

316. Walsh D., Furuzono T., Tanaka J., Preparation of porous composite implant materials by *in situ* polymerization of porous apatite containing ε-caprolactone or methyl methacrylate. *Biomaterials*, (2001), 22, 1205–1212.

317. Kim H.W., Biomedical nanocomposites of hydroxyapatite/polycaprolactone obtained by surfactant mediation. *J. Biomed. Mater. Res. A*, (2007), 83A, 169–177.

318. Heo S.J., Kim S.E., Wei J., Hyun Y.T., Yun H.S., Kim D.H., Shin J.W., Shin J.W., Fabrication and characterization of novel nano- and micro-HA/PCL composite scaffolds using a modified rapid prototyping process. *J. Biomed. Mater. Res. A*, (2009), 89A, 108–116.

319. Chuenjitkuntaworn B., Inrung W., Damrongsri D., Mekaapiruk K., Supaphol P., Pavasant P., Polycaprolactone/hydroxyapatite composite scaffolds: preparation, characterization, and *in vitro* and *in vivo* biological responses of human primary bone cells. *J. Biomed. Mater. Res. A*, (2010), 94A, 241–251.

320. Bang L.T., Kawachi G., Nakagawa M., Munar M., Ishikawa K., Othman R., The use of poly (ε-caprolactone) to enhance the mechanical strength of porous Si-substituted carbonate apatite. *J. Appl. Polym. Sci.*, (2013), 130, 426–433.

321. Mohd Yusoff M.F., Abdul Kadir M.R., Iqbal N., Hassan M.A., Hussain R., Dipcoating of poly (ε-caprolactone)/hydroxyapatite composite coating on Ti6Al4V for enhanced corrosion protection. *Surf. Coat. Technol.*, (2014), 245, 102–107.

322. Kim B.S., Yang S.S., Lee J., A polycaprolactone/cuttlefish bone-derived hydroxyapatite composite porous scaffold for bone tissue engineering. *J. Biomed. Mater. Res. B Appl. Biomater.*, (2014), 102B, 943–951.

323. Hajiali F., Tajbakhsh S., Shojaei A., Fabrication and properties of polycaprolactone composites containing calcium phosphate-based ceramics and bioactive glasses in bone tissue engineering: a review. *Polym. Rev.*, (2017), 58, 164–207.

324. Huang B., Caetano G., Vyas C., Blaker J.J., Diver C., Bártolo P. Polymer-ceramic, composite scaffolds: the effect of hydroxyapatite and β-tri-calcium phosphate. *Materials*, (2018), 11, 129.

325. Causa F., Netti P.A., Ambrosio L., Ciapetti G., Baldini N., Pagani S., Martini D., Giunti A., Poly-ε-caprolactone/hydroxyapatite composites for bone regeneration: *in vitro* characterization and human osteoblast response. *J. Biomed. Mater. Res. A*, (2006), 76A, 151–162.

326. Thomas V., Jagani S., Johnson K., Jose M.V., Dean D.R., Vohra Y.K., Nyairo E., Electrospun bioactive nanocomposite scaffolds of polycaprolactone and nanohydroxyapatite for bone tissue engineering. *J. Nanosci. Nanotechol.*, (2006), 6, 487–493.

327. Marra K.G., Szem J.W., Kumta P.N., DiMilla P.A., Weiss L.E., *In vitro* analysis of biodegradable polymer blend/hydroxyapatite composites for bone tissue engineering. *J. Biomed. Mater. Res.*, (1999), 47, 324–335.

328. Dunn A., Campbell P., Marra K.G., The influence of polymer blend composition on the degradation of polymer/hydroxyapatite biomaterials. *J. Mater. Sci. Mater. Med.*, (2001), 12, 673–677.

329. Calandrelli L., Immirzi B., Malinconico M., Volpe M., Oliva A., Ragione F., Preparation and characterization of composites based on biodegradable polymers for *in vivo* application. *Polymer*, (2000), 41, 8027–8033.

330. Chen B., Sun K., Poly(ε-caprolactone)/hydroxyapatite composites: effects of particle size, molecular weight distribution and irradiation on interfacial interaction and properties. *Polym. Test.*, (2005), 24, 64–70.

331. Kim H.W., Knowles J.C., Kim H.E., Hydroxyapatite/poly(ε-caprolactone) composite coatings on hydroxyapatite porous bone scaffold for drug delivery. *Biomaterials*, (2004), 25, 1279–1287.

332. Ural E., Kesenci K., Fambri L., Migliaresi C., Piskin E., Poly(D,L-lactide/ε-caprolactone)/hydroxyapatite composites. *Biomaterials*, (2000), 21, 2147–2154.

333. Rodenas-Rochina J., Vidaurre A., Cortázar I.C., Lebourg M., Effects of hydroxyapatite filler on long-term hydrolytic degradation of PLLA/PCL porous scaffolds. *Polym. Degrad. Stabil.*, (2015), 119, 121–131.

334. Kim H.W., Lee E.J., Kim H.E., Salih V., Knowles J.C., Effect of fluoridation of hydroxyapatite in hydroxyapatite/polycaprolactone composites on osteoblast activity. *Biomaterials*, (2005), 26, 4395–4404.

335. Gloria A., Russo T., D'Amora U., Zeppetelli S., D'Alessandro T., Sandri M., Bañobre-López M., Piñeiro-Redondo Y., Uhlarz M., Tampieri A., Rivas J., Herrmannsdörfer T., Dediu V.A., Ambrosio L., de Santis R., Magnetic poly(ε-caprolactone)/iron-doped hydroxyapatite nanocomposite substrates for advanced bone tissue engineering. *J. R. Soc. Interface*, (2013), 10, 20120833.

336. Shokrollahi P., Mirzadeh H., Scherman O.A., Huck W.T.S., Biological and mechanical properties of novel composites based on supramolecular polycaprolactone and functionalized hydroxyapatite. *J. Biomed. Mater. Res. A*, (2010), 95A, 209–221.

337. Mehmanchi M., Shokrollahi P., Atai M., Omidian H., Bagheri R., Supramolecular polycaprolactone nanocomposite based on functionalized hydroxyapatite. *J. Bioact. Compat. Polym.*, (2012), 27, 467–480.

338. Yu J., Xu Y., Li S., Seifert G.V., Becker M.L., Three-dimensional printing of nano hydroxyapatite/poly(ester urea) composite scaffolds with enhanced bioactivity. *Biomacromolecules*, (2017), 18, 4171–4183.

339. Deng C., Wang B., Dongqin X., Zhou S., Duan K., Weng J., Preparation and shape memory property of hydroxyapatite/poly (vinyl alcohol) composite. *Polym. – Plast. Technol. Eng.*, (2012), 51, 1315–1318.

340. Kutikov A.B., Reyer K.A., Song J., Shape-memory performance of thermoplastic amphiphilic triblock copolymer poly(D,L-lactic acid-co-ethylene glycol-co-D,L-lactic acid) (PELA)/hydroxyapatite composites. *Macromol. Chem. Phys.*, (2014), 215, 2482–2490.

341. Wong T.W., Wahit M.U., Abdul Kadir M.R., Soheilmoghaddam M., Balakrishnan H., A novel poly(xylitol-co-dodecanedioate)/hydroxyapatite composite with shape-memory behaviour. *Mater. Lett.*, (2014), 126, 105–108.

342. Behl M., Razzaq M.Y., Lendlein A., Multifunctional shape-memory polymers. *Adv. Mater.*, (2010), 22, 3388–3410.

343. Wang R., Sun K., Wang J., He Y., Song P., Xiong Y., Preparation and application of natural polymer/hydroxyapatite composite. *Prog. Chem.*, (2016), 28, 885–895.

344. Ramesh N., Moratti S.C., Dias G.J., Hydroxyapatite-polymer biocomposites for bone regeneration: a review of current trends. *J. Biomed. Mater. Res. B Appl. Biomater.*, (2018), 106, 2046–2057.

345. Handschel J., Wiesmann H.P., Stratmann U., Kleinheinz J., Meyer U., Joos U., TCP is hardly resorbed and not osteoconductive in a non-loading calvarial model. *Biomaterials*, (2002), 23, 1689–1695.

346. Kikuchi M., Tanaka J., Chemical interaction in β-tricalcium phosphate/copolymerized poly-L-lactide composites. *J. Ceram. Soc. Jpn.*, (2000), 108, 642–645.

347. Aunoble S., Clement D., Frayssinet P., Harmand M.F., le Huec J.C., Biological performance of a new β-TCP/PLLA composite material for applications in spine surgery: *in vitro* and *in vivo* studies. *J. Biomed. Mater. Res. A*, (2006), 78A, 416–422.

348. Haaparanta A.M., Haimi S., Ellä, V., Hopper N., Miettinen S., Suuronen R., Kellomäki M., Porous polylactide/β-tricalcium phosphate composite scaffolds for tissue engineering applications. *J. Tissue Eng. Regen. Med.*, (2010), 4, 366–373.

349. Shin D.Y., Kang M.H., Kang I.G., Kim H.E., Jeong S.H., *In vitro* and *in vivo* evaluation of polylactic acid-based composite with tricalcium phosphate microsphere for enhanced biodegradability and osseointegration. *J. Biomater. Appl.*, (2018), 32, 1360–1370.

350. Kikuchi M., Koyama Y., Yamada T., Imamura Y., Okada T., Shirahama N., Akita K., Takakuda K., Tanaka J., Development of guided bone regeneration membrane composed of β-tricalcium phosphate and poly(L-lactide-*co*-glycolide-*co*-ε-caprolactone) composites. *Biomaterials*, (2004), 25, 5979–5986.

351. Chen T.M., Yao C.H., Wang H.J., Chou G.H., Lee T.W., Lin F.H., Evaluation of a novel malleable, biodegradable osteoconductive composite in a rabbit cranial defect model. *Mater. Chem. Phys.*, (1998), 55, 44–50.

352. Dong G.C., Chen H.M., Yao C.H., A novel bone substitute composite composed of tricalcium phosphate, gelatin and drynaria fortunei herbal extract. *J. Biomed. Mater. Res. A*, (2008), 84A, 167–177.

353. Ji J., Yuan X., Xia Z., Liu P., Chen J., Porous β-tricalcium phosphate composite scaffold reinforced by K_2HPO_4 and gelatin. *Key Eng. Mater.*, (2010), 434–435, 620–623.

354. Yao C.H., Liu B.S., Hsu S.H., Chen Y.S., Tsai C.C., Biocompatibility and biodegradation of a bone composite containing tricalcium phosphate and genipin crosslinked gelatin. *J. Biomed. Mater. Res. A*, (2004), 69A, 709–717.

355. Eslaminejad M.B., Mirzadeh H., Mohamadi Y., Nickmahzar A., Bone differentiation of marrow-derived mesenchymal stem cells using β-tricalcium phosphate-alginate-gelatin hybrid scaffolds. *J. Tissue Eng. Regen. Med.*, (2007), 1, 417–424.

356. Takahashi Y., Yamamoto M., Tabata Y., Osteogenic differentiation of mesenchymal stem cells in biodegradable sponges composed of gelatin and β-tricalcium phosphate. *Biomaterials*, (2005), 26, 3587–3596.

357. Bigi A., Cantelli I., Panzavolta S., Rubini K., α-Tricalcium phosphate-gelatin composite cements. *J. Appl. Biomater. Biomech.*, (2004), 2, 81–87.

358. Yang S.H., Hsu C.K., Wang K.C., Hou S.M., Lin F.H., Tricalcium phosphate and glutaraldehyde crosslinked gelatin incorporating bone morphogenetic protein – a viable scaffold for bone tissue engineering. *J. Biomed. Mater. Res. B Appl. Biomater.*, (2005), 74B, 468–475.

359. Kato M., Namikawa T., Terai H., Hoshino M., Miyamoto S., Takaoka K., Ectopic bone formation in mice associated with a lactic acid/dioxanone/ ethylene glycol copolymer-tricalcium phosphate composite with added recombinant human bone morphogenetic protein-2. *Biomaterials*, (2006), 27, 3927–3933.

360. Muramatsu K., Oba K., Mukai D., Hasegawa K., Masuda S., Yoshihara Y., Subacute systemic toxicity assessment of β-tricalcium phosphate/ carboxymethyl-chitin composite implanted in rat femur. *J. Mater. Sci. Mater. Med.*, (2007), 18, 513–522.

361. Panzavolta S., Fini M., Nicoletti A., Bracci B., Rubini K., Giardino R., Bigi A., Porous composite scaffolds based on gelatin and partially hydrolyzed α-tricalcium phosphate. *Acta Biomater.*, (2009), 5, 636–643.

362. Uchino T., Kamitakahara M., Otsuka M., Ohtsuki C., Hydroxyapatite-forming capability and mechanical properties of organic-inorganic hybrids and α-tricalcium phosphate porous bodies. *J. Ceram. Soc. Jpn.*, (2010), 118, 57–61.

363. Boguń, M., Rabiej S., The influence of fiber formation conditions on the structure and properties of nanocomposite alginate fibers containing tricalcium phosphate or montmorillonite. *Polym. Composite*, (2010), 31, 1321–1331.

364. Park C.H., Kim E.K., Tijing L.D., Amarjargal A., Pant H.R., Kim C.S., Shon H.K., Preparation and characterization of LA/PCL composite fibers containing beta tricalcium phosphate (β-TCP) particles. *Ceram. Int.*, (2014), 40, 5049–5054.

365. Ngamviriyavong P., Patntirapong S., Janvikul W., Arphavasin S., Meesap P., Singhatanadgit W., Development of poly(butylene succinate)/calcium phosphate composites for bone engineering. *Compos. Interface*, (2014), 21, 431–441.

366. Flauder S., Sajzew R., Müller F.A., Mechanical properties of porous β-tricalcium phosphate composites prepared by ice-templating and poly(σ-caprolactone) impregnation. *ACS Appl. Mater. Interf.*, (2015), 7, 845–851.

367. Agyemang F.O., Sheikh F.A., Appiah-Ntiamoah R., Chandradass J., Kim H., Synthesis and characterization of poly (vinylidene fluoride)–calcium phosphate composite for potential tissue engineering applications. *Ceram. Int.*, (2015), 41, 7066–7072.

368. Cohen B., Panker M., Zuckerman E., Foox M., Zilberman M., Effect of calcium phosphate-based fillers on the structure and bonding strength of novel gelatin-alginate bioadhesives. *J. Biomater. Appl.*, (2014), 28, 1366–1375.

369. Bleach N.C., Tanner K.E., Kellomäki M., Törmälä, P., Effect of filler type on the mechanical properties of self-reinforced polylactide-calcium phosphate composites. *J. Mater. Sci. Mater. Med.*, (2001), 12, 911–915.

370. Liu L., Xiong Z., Yan Y.N., Hu Y.Y., Zhang R.J., Wang S.G., Porous morphology, porosity, mechanical properties of poly(α-hydroxy acid)-tricalcium phosphate composite scaffolds fabricated by low-temperature deposition. *J. Biomed. Mater. Res. A*, (2007), 82A, 618–629.

371. Zhang Y., Zhang M.Q., Synthesis and characterization of macroporous chitosan/calcium phosphate composite scaffolds for tissue engineering. *J. Biomed. Mater. Res.*, (2001), 55, 304–312.

372. Rai B., Teoh S.H., Hutmacher D.W., Cao T., Ho K.H., Novel PCL-based honeycomb scaffolds as drug delivery systems for rhBMP-2. *Biomaterials*, (2005), 26, 3739–3748.

373. Rai B., Teoh S.H., Ho K.H., Hutmacher D.W., Cao T., Chen F., Yacob K., The effect of rhBMP-2 on canine osteoblasts seeded onto 3D bioactive polycaprolactone scaffolds. *Biomaterials*, (2004), 25, 5499–5506.

374. Lei Y., Rai B., Ho K.H., Teoh S.H., *In vitro* degradation of novel bioactive polycaprolactone – 20% tricalcium phosphate composite scaffolds for bone engineering. *Mater. Sci. Eng. C*, (2007), 27, 293–298.

375. Miyai T., Ito A., Tamazawa G., Matsuno T., Sogo Y., Nakamura C., Yamazaki A., Satoh T., Antibiotic-loaded poly-ε-caprolactone and porous β-tricalcium phosphate composite for treating osteomyelitis. *Biomaterials*, (2008), 29, 350–358.

376. Li Y., Wu Z.G., Li X.K., Guo Z., Wu S.H., Zhang Y.Q., Shi L., Teoh S.H., Liu Y.C., Zhang Z.Y., A polycaprolactone-tricalcium phosphate composite scaffold as an autograft-free spinal fusion cage in a sheep model. *Biomaterials*, (2014), 35, 5647–5659.

377. Takahashi Y., Yamamoto M., Tabata Y., Enhanced osteoinduction by controlled release of bone morphogenetic protein-2 from biodegradable sponge composed of gelatin and β-tricalcium phosphate. *Biomaterials*, (2005), 26, 4856–4865.

378. Ignatius A.A., Betz O., Augat P., Claes L.E., *In vivo* investigations on composites made of resorbable ceramics and poly(lactide) used as bone graft substitutes. *J. Biomed. Mater. Res. Appl. Biomater.*, (2001), 58, 701–709.

379. Miao X., Lim W.K., Huang X., Chen Y., Preparation and characterization of interpenetrating phased TCP/HA/PLGA composites. *Mater. Lett.*, (2005), 59, 4000–4005.

380. Ozbek B., Erdogan B., Ekren N., Oktar F.N., Akyol S., Ben-Nissan B., Sasmazel H.T., Kalkandelen C., Mergen A., Kuruca S.E., Ozen G., Gunduz O., Production of the novel fibrous structure of poly(ε-caprolactone)/tricalcium phosphate/hexagonal boron nitride composites for bone tissue engineering. *J. Austral. Ceram. Soc.*, (2018), 54, 251–260.

381. Dorozhkin S.V., Multiphasic calcium orthophosphate (CaPO₄) bioceramics and their biomedical applications. *Ceram. Int.*, (2016), 42, 6529–6554.

382. Brodie J.C., Goldie E., Connel G., Merry J., Grant M.H., Osteoblast interactions with calcium phosphate ceramics modified by coating with type I collagen. *J. Biomed. Mater. Res. A*, (2005), 73A, 409–421.

383. Zhang L.F., Sun R., Xu L., Du J., Xiong Z.C., Chen H.C., Xiong C.D., Hydrophilic poly (ethylene glycol) coating on PDLLA/BCP bone scaffold for drug delivery and cell culture. *Mater. Sci. Eng. C*, (2008), 28, 141–149.

384. Ignjatovic N., Ninkov P., Ajdukovic Z., Konstantinovic V., Uskokovic D., Biphasic calcium phosphate/poly-(D,L-lactide-co-glycolide) biocomposite as filler and blocks for reparation of bone tissue. *Mater. Sci. Forum*, (2005), 494, 519–524.

385. Ignjatovic N., Ninkov P., Ajdukovic Z., Vasiljevic-Radovic D., Uskokovic D., Biphasic calcium phosphate coated with poly-D,L-lactide-co-glycolide biomaterial as a bone substitute. *J. Eur. Ceram. Soc.*, (2007), 27, 1589–1594.

386. Yang W., Yin G., Zhou D., Gu J., Li Y., *In vitro* characteristics of surface-modified biphasic calcium phosphate/poly(L-Lactide) biocomposite. *Adv. Eng. Mater.*, (2010), 12, B128–B132.

387. Ignjatovic N., Ninkov P., Kojic V., Bokurov M., Srdic V., Krnojelac D., Selakovic S., Uskokovic D., Cytotoxicity and fibroblast properties during *in vitro* test of biphasic calcium phosphate/poly-D,L-lactide-co-glycolide biocomposites and different phosphate materials. *Microsc. Res. Techniq.*, (2006), 69, 976–982.

388. Ajdukovic Z., Ignjatovic N., Petrovic D., Uskokovic D., Substitution of osteoporotic alveolar bone by biphasic calcium phosphate/poly-D,L-lactide-co-glycolide biomaterials. *J. Biomater. Appl.*, (2007), 21, 317–328.

389. Kim H.W., Knowles J.C., Kim H.E., Effect of biphasic calcium phosphates on drug release and biological and mechanical properties of poly(ε-caprolactone) composite membranes. *J. Biomed. Mater. Res. A*, (2004), 70A, 467–479.

390. Kwak K.A., Jyoti M.A., Song H.Y., *In vitro* and *in vivo* studies of three dimensional porous composites of biphasic calcium phosphate/poly ε-caprolactone: effect of bio-functionalization for bone tissue engineering. *Appl. Surf. Sci.*, (2014), 301, 307–314.

391. van Leeuwen A.C., Yuan H., Passanisi G., van der Meer J.W., de Bruijn J.D., van Kooten T.G., Grijpma D.W., Bos R.R., Poly(trimethylene carbonate) and biphasic calcium phosphate composites for orbital floor reconstruction: a feasibility study in sheep. *Eur. Cell. Mater.*, (2014), 27, 81–96, discussion 96–97.

392. Bakhtiari L., Rezai H.R., Hosseinalipour S.M., Shokrgozar M.A., Investigation of biphasic calcium phosphate/gelatin nanocomposite scaffolds as a bone tissue engineering. *Ceram. Int.*, (2010), 36, 2421–2426.

393. Bakhtiari L., Rezai H.R., Hosseinalipour S.M., Shokrgozar M.A., Preparation of porous Biphasic calcium phosphate-gelatin nanocomposite for bone tissue engineering. *J. Nano Res.*, (2010), 11, 67–72.

394. Matsuda A., Ikoma T., Kobayashi H., Tanaka J., Preparation and mechanical property of core-shell type chitosan/calcium phosphate composite fiber. *Mater. Sci. Eng. C*, (2004), 24, 723–728.

395. Rattanachan S., Lorprayoon C., Boonphayak P., Synthesis of chitosan/brushite powders for bone cement composites. *J. Ceram. Soc. Jpn.*, (2008), 116, 36–41.

396. Ohsawa H., Ito A., Sogo Y., Yamazaki A., Ohno T., Synthesis of albumin/DCP nano-composite particles. *Key Eng. Mater.*, (2007), 330–332, 239–242.

397. Mohammad F., Arfin T., Al-Lohedan H.A., Synthesis, characterization and applications of ethyl cellulose-based polymeric calcium (II) hydrogen phosphate composite. *J. Electron. Mater.*, (2018), 47, 2954–2963.

398. Xu H.H.K., Sun L., Weir M.D., Antonucci J.M., Takagi S., Chow L.C., Peltz M., Nano DCPA-whisker composites with high strength and Ca and PO_4 release. *J. Dent. Res.*, (2006), 85, 722–727.

399. Xu H.H.K., Weir M.D., Sun L., Takagi S., Chow L.C., Effects of calcium phosphate nanoparticles on Ca-PO_4 composite. *J. Dent. Res.*, (2007), 86, 378–383.

400. Xu H.H.K., Weir M.D., Sun L., Nanocomposites with Ca and PO_4 release: effects of reinforcement, dicalcium phosphate particle size and silanization. *Dent. Mater.*, (2007), 23, 1482–1491.

401. Chen W.C., Chang K.C., Wu H.Y., Ko C.L., Huang C.L., Thermal cycling effect of dicalcium phosphate-reinforced composites on auto-mineralized dental resin. *Mater. Sci. Eng. C*, (2014), 45, 359–368.

402. El-Meliegy E., Mabrouk M., Kamal G.M., Awad S.M., El-Tohamy A.M., El Gohary M.I., Anticancer drug carriers using dicalcium phosphate/dextran/CMCnanocomposite scaffolds. *J. Drug Delivery Sci. Technol.*, (2018), 45, 315–322.

403. Tortet L., Gavarri J.R., Nihoul G., Dianoux A.J., Proton mobilities in brushite and brushite/polymer composites. *Solid State Ionics*, (1997), 97, 253–256.

404. Tortet L., Gavarri J.R., Musso J., Nihoul G., Sarychev A.K., Percolation and modeling of proton conduction in polymer/brushite composites. *J. Solid State Chem.*, (1998), 141, 392–403.

405. Dorozhkin S.V., Amorphous calcium orthophosphates: nature, chemistry and biomedical applications. *Int. J. Mater. Chem.*, (2012), 2, 19–46.

406. Dorozhkin S.V., Calcium orthophosphates ($CaPO_4$) and dentistry. *Bioceram. Dev. Appl.*, (2016), 6, 96 (28 pages).

407. Zhang L., Weir M.D., Chow L.C., Antonucci J.M., Chen J., Xu H.H.K., Novel rechargeable calcium phosphate dental nanocomposite. *Dent. Mater.*, (2016), 32, 285–293.

408. Zhang L., Weir M.D., Chow L.C., Reynolds M.A., Xu H.H.K., Rechargeable calcium phosphate orthodontic cement with sustained ion release and re-release. *Sci. Rep.*, (2016), 6, 36476 (11 pages).

409. Xie X.J., Xing D., Wang L., Zhou H., Weir M.D., Bai Y.X., Xu H.H.K., Novel rechargeable calcium phosphate nanoparticle-containing orthodontic cement. *Int. J. Oral Sci.*, (2018), 9, 24–32.

410. Liang K., Xiao S., Wu J., Li J., Weir M.D., Cheng L., Reynolds M.A., Zhou X., Xu H.H.K., Long-term dentin remineralization by poly(amido amine) and rechargeable calcium phosphate nanocomposite after fluid challenges. *Dent. Mater.*, (2018), 34, 607–618.

411. Gutierrez M.C., Jobbágy M., Ferrer M.L., del Monte F., Enzymatic synthesis of amorphous calcium phosphate-chitosan nanocomposites and their processing into hierarchical structures. *Chem. Mater.*, (2008), 20, 11–13.

412. Hakimimehr D., Liu D.M., Troczynski T., *In-situ* preparation of poly(propylene fumarate) – hydroxyapatite composite. *Biomaterials*, (2005), 26, 7297–7303.

413. Antonucci J.M., Regnault W.F., Skrtic D., Polymerization shrinkage and stress development in amorphous calcium phosphate/urethane dimethacrylate polymeric composites. *J. Compos. Mater.*, (2010), 44, 355–367.

414. Wang K.W., Zhu Y.J., Chen F., Cao S.W., Calcium phosphate/block copolymer hybrid porous nanospheres: preparation and application in drug delivery. *Mater. Lett.*, (2010), 64, 2299–2301.

415. Cao S.W., Zhu Y.J., Wu J., Wang K.W., Tang Q.L., Preparation and sustained-release property of triblock copolymer/calcium phosphate nanocomposite as nanocarrier for hydrophobic drug. *Nanoscale Res. Lett.*, (2010), 5, 781–785.

416. Iwama R., Anada T., Shiwaku Y., Tsuchiya K., Takahashi T., Suzuki O., Osteogenic cellular activity around onlaid octacalcium phosphate-gelatin composite onto rat calvaria. *J. Biomed. Mater. Res. A*, (2018), 106A, 1322–1333.

417. Suzuki O., Octacalcium phosphate (OCP)-based bone substitute materials. *Jpn. Dent. Sci. Rev.*, (2013), 49, 58–71.

418. Gelse K., Pöschl E., Aigner T., Collagens – structure, function, and biosynthesis. *Adv. Drug Deliv. Rev.*, (2003), 55, 1531–1546.

419. Fratzl P. (ed.), *Collagen: Structure and Mechanics*, Springer: New York, 2010, p. 510.

420. Tsai C.H., Chou M.Y., Jonas M., Tien Y.T., Chi E.Y., A composite graft material containing bone particles and collagen in osteoinduction in mouse. *J. Biomed. Mater. Res.*, (2002), 63, 65–70.

421. Xie J., Baumann M.J., McCabe L.R., Osteoblasts respond to hydroxyapatite surfaces with immediate changes in gene expression. *J. Biomed. Mater. Res. A*, (2004), 71A, 108–117.

422. Tcacencu I., Wendel M., Collagen-hydroxyapatite composite enhances regeneration of calvaria bone defects in young rats but postpones the regeneration of calvaria bone in aged rats. *J. Mater. Sci. Mater. Med.*, (2008), 19, 2015–2021.

423. Yamauchi K., Goda T., Takeuchi N., Einaga H., Tanabe T., Preparation of collagen/calcium phosphate multilayer sheet using enzymatic mineralization. *Biomaterials*, (2004), 25, 5481–5489.

424. Liu C. Collagen–hydroxyapatite composite scaffolds for tissue engineering. In: *Hydroxyapatite (HAp) for Biomedical Applications*, Mucalo M.R. (ed.), Woodhead publishing series in biomaterials: Number 95, Elsevier: Cambridge, UK, 2015, pp. 211–234.

425. Hellmich C., Ulm F.J., Are mineralized tissues open crystal foams reinforced by crosslinked collagen? – Some energy arguments. *J. Biomech.*, (2002), 35, 1199–1212.

426. Roveri N., Falini G., Sidoti M.C., Tampieri A., Landi E., Sandri M., Parma B., Biologically inspired growth of hydroxyapatite nanocrystals inside self-assembled collagen fibers. *Mater. Sci. Eng. C*, (2003), 23, 441–446.

427. Tampieri A., Celotti G., Landi E., From biomimetic apatites to biologically inspired composites. *Anal. Bioanal. Chem.*, (2005), 381, 568–576.

428. Tampieri, A., Celotti G., Landi E., Sandri M., Roveri N., Falini G., Biologically inspired synthesis of bone-like composite: self-assembled collagen fibers/hydroxyapatite nanocrystals. *J. Biomed. Mater. Res. A,* (2003), 67A, 618–625.

429. Clarke K.I., Graves S.E., Wong A.T.C., Triffit J.T., Francis M.J.O., Czernuszka J.T., Investigation into the formation and mechanical properties of a bioactive material based on collagen and calcium phosphate. *J. Mater. Sci. Mater. Med.*, (1993), 4, 107–110.

430. Ten Huisen K.S., Martin R.I., Klimkiewicz M., Brown P.W., Formation and properties of a synthetic bone composite: hydroxyapatite-collagen. *J. Biomed. Mater. Res.*, (1995), 29, 803–810.

431. Ishikawa H., Koshino T., Takeuchi R., Saito T., Effects of collagen gel mixed with hydroxyapatite power on interface between newly formed bone and grafted Achilles tendon in rabbit femoral bone tunnel. *Biomaterials,* (2001), 22, 1689–1694.

432. Ltoh S., Kikuchi M., Takakuda K., Koyama Y., Matsumoto H.N., Ichinose S., Tanaka J., Kawauchi T., Shinomiya K., The biocompatibility and osteoconductive activity of a novel hydroxyapatite/collagen composite biomaterial and its function as a carrier of rhBMP-2. *J. Biomed. Mater. Res.*, (2001), 54, 445–453.

433. Uskokovic V., Ignjatovic N., Petranovic N., Synthesis and characterization of hydroxyapatite-collagen biocomposite materials. *Mater. Sci. Forum,* (2002), 413, 269–274.

434. Yoon B.H., Kim H.W., Lee S.H., Bae C.J., Koh Y.H., Kong Y.M., Kim H.E., Stability and cellular responses to fluorapatite-collagen composites. *Biomaterials,* (2005), 26, 2957–2963.

435. Wahl D.A., Czernuszka J.T., Collagen-hydroxyapatite composites for hard tissue repair. *Eur. Cell Mater.*, (2006), 11, 43–56.

436. Sachlos E., Gotora D., Czernuszka J.T., Collagen scaffolds reinforced with biomimetic composite nano-sized carbonate-substituted hydroxyapatite crystals and shaped by rapid prototyping to contain internal microchannels. *Tissue Eng.*, (2006), 12, 2479–2487.

437. Teng S.H., Lee E.J., Park C.S., Choi W.Y., Shin D.S., Kim H.E., Bioactive nanocomposite coatings of collagen/hydroxyapatite on titanium substrates. *J. Mater. Sci. Mater. Med.*, (2008), 19, 2453–2461.

438. Song J.H., Kim H.E., Kim H.W., Collagen-apatite nanocomposite membranes for guided bone regeneration. *J. Biomed. Mater. Res. B Appl. Biomater.*, (2007), 83B, 248–257.

439. Pek Y.S., Gao S., Arshad M.S.M., Leck K.J., Ying J.Y., Porous collagen-apatite nanocomposite foams as bone regeneration scaffolds. *Biomaterials,* (2008), 29, 4300–4305.

440. Zhao H., Huang C., Jin H., Cai J., A novel route for collagen/hydroxyapatite preparation by enzymatic decomposition of urea. *J. Compos. Mater.*, (2010), 44, 2127–2133.

441. Kozłowska J., Sionkowska A., Effects of different crosslinking methods on the properties of collagen-calcium phosphate composite materials. *Int. J. Biol. Macromol.*, (2015), 74, 397–403.

442. Banglmaier R.F., Sander E.A., VandeVord P.J., Induction and quantification of collagen fiber alignment in a three-dimensional hydroxyapatite-collagen composite scaffold. *Acta Biomater.*, (2015), 17, 26–35.

443. Banks E., Nakajima S., Shapiro L.C., Tilevitz O., Alonzo J.R., Chianelli R.R., Fibrous apatite grown on modified collagen. *Science*, (1977), 198, 1164–1166.

444. Hayashi K., Yabuki T., Tabuchi K., Fujii T., Repair of experimental bone defect with a collagen block containing synthesized apatite. *Arch. Orthop. Traum. Surg.*, (1982), 99, 265–269.

445. Mittelmeier H., Nizzard M., Knochenregeneration mit industriell gefertigtem Collagen Apatit Implantat ("Collapat"). In: *Osteogenese und Knochenwachstum*, Hackenbroch M.H., Refior H.J., Jäger M.G. (eds), Thieme: Stuttgart, Germany, 1982, pp. 194–197.

446. Serre C.M., Papillard M., Chavassieux P., Boivin G., *In vitro* induction of a calcifying matrix by biomaterials constituted of collagen and/or hydroxyapatite: an ultrastructural comparison of three types of biomaterials. *Biomaterials*, (1993), 14, 97–106.

447. Scabbia A., Trombelli L., A comparative study on the use of a HA/collagen/chondroitin sulphate biomaterial (Biostite®) and a bovine-derived HA xenograft (Bio-Oss®) in the treatment of deep intraosseous defects. *J. Clin. Periodontol.*, (2004), 31, 348–355.

448. Yamasaki Y., Yoshida Y., Okazaki M., Shimazu A., Kubo T., Akagawa Y., Uchida T., Action of FGMgCO$_3$Ap-collagen composite in promoting bone formation. *Biomaterials*, (2003), 24, 4913–4920.

449. Wang X., Grogan S.P., Rieser F., Winkelmann V., Maquet V., Berge M.L., Mainil-Varlet P., Tissue engineering of biphasic cartilage constructs using various biodegradable scaffolds: an *in vitro* study. *Biomaterials*, (2004), 25, 3681–3688.

450. Zahn D., Multi-scale simulations of apatite–collagen composites: from molecules to materials. *Front. Mater. Sci.*, (2017), 11, 1–12.

451. Chang M.C., Ikoma T., Kikuchi M., Tanaka J., The cross-linkage effect of hydroxyapatite/collagen nanocomposites on a self-organization phenomenon. *J. Mater. Sci. Mater. Med.*, (2002), 13, 993–997.

452. Iijima M., Moriwaki Y., Kuboki Y., Oriented growth of octacalcium phosphate on and inside the collagenous matrix *in vitro*. *Connect. Tissue Res.*, (1996), 32, 519–524.

453. Miyamoto Y., Ishikawa K., Takechi M., Toh T., Yuasa T., Nagayama M., Suzuki K., Basic properties of calcium phosphate cement containing atelocollagen in its liquid or powder phases. *Biomaterials*, (1998), 19, 707–715.

454. Iijima M., Moriwaki Y., Kuboki Y., *In vitro* crystal growth of octacalcium phosphate on type I collagen fiber. *J. Cryst. Growth*, (1994), 137, 553–560.
455. Iijima M., Iijima K., Moriwaki Y., Kuboki Y., Oriented growth of octacalcium phosphate crystals on type I collagen fibrils under physiological conditions. *J. Cryst. Growth*, (1994), 140, 91–99.
456. Lawson A.C., Czernuszka J.T., Collagen – calcium phosphate composites. *Proc. Inst. Mech. Eng. H*, (1998), 212, 413–425.
457. Du C., Cui F.Z., Zhang W., Feng Q.L., Zhu X.D., de Groot K., Formation of calcium phosphate/collagen composites through mineralization of collagen matrix. *J. Biomed. Mater. Res.*, (2000), 50, 518–527.
458. Kamakura S., Sasaki K., Honda Y., Anada T., Suzuki O., Octacalcium phosphate combined with collagen orthotopically enhances bone regeneration. *J. Biomed. Mater. Res. B Appl. Biomater.*, (2006), 79B, 210–217.
459. Kawai T., Anada T., Honda Y., Kamakura S., Matsui K., Matsui A., Sasaki K., Morimoto S., Echigo S., Suzuki O., Synthetic octacalcium phosphate augments bone regeneration correlated with its content in collagen scaffold. *Tissue Eng. A*, (2009), 15, 23–32.
460. Masuda T., Kawai T., Anada T., Kamakura S., Suzuki O., Quality of regenerated bone enhanced by implantation of octacalcium phosphate-collagen composite. *Tissue Eng. C*, (2010), 16, 471–478.
461. Kikuchi M., Ikoma T., Itoh S., Matsumoto H.N., Koyama Y., Takakuda K., Shinomiya K., Tanaka J., Biomimetic synthesis of bone-like nanocomposites using the self-organization mechanism of hydroxyapatite and collagen. *Compos. Sci. Technol.*, (2004), 64, 819–825.
462. Yunoki S., Ikoma T., Monkawal A., Ohtal K., Tanaka J., Preparation and characterization of hydroxyapatite/collagen nanocomposite gel. *J. Nanosci. Nanotechnol.*, (2007), 7, 818–821.
463. Li X., Chang J., Preparation of bone-like apatite-collagen nanocomposites by a biomimetic process with phosphorylated collagen. *J. Biomed. Mater. Res. A*, (2008), 85A, 293–300.
464. Ficai A., Andronescu E., Voicu G., Ghitulica C., Vasile B.S., Ficai D., Trandafir V., Self-assembled collagen/hydroxyapatite composite materials. *Chem. Eng. J.*, (2010), 160, 794–800.
465. Jee S.S., Thula T.T., Gower L.B., Development of bone-like composites via the polymer-induced liquid-precursor (PILP) process. Part 1: Influence of polymer molecular weight. *Acta Biomater.*, (2010), 6, 3676–3686.
466. Kane R.J., Weiss-Bilka H.E., Meagher M.J., Liu Y., Gargac J.A., Niebur G.L., Wagner D.R., Roeder R.K., Hydroxyapatite reinforced collagen scaffolds with improved architecture and mechanical properties. *Acta Biomater.*, (2015), 17, 16–25.
467. Bu H., Li G., Comparative investigation of hydroxyapatite/collagen composites prepared by $CaCl_2$ addition at different time points in collagen self-assembly process. *J. Mater. Sci.*, (2018), 53, 6313–6324.

468. Andronescu E., Ficai M., Voicu G., Ficai D., Maganu M., Ficai A., Synthesis and characterization of collagen/hydroxyapatite: magnetite composite material for bone cancer treatment. *J. Mater. Sci. Mater. Med.*, (2010), 21, 2237–2242.

469. Ficai M., Andronescu E., Ficai D., Voicu G., Ficai A., Synthesis and characterization of COLL-PVA/HA hybrid materials with stratified morphology. *Colloid Surface B*, (2010), 81, 614–619.

470. Inzana J.A., Olvera D., Fuller S.M., Kelly J.P., Graeve O.A., Schwarz E.M., Kates S.L., Awad H.A., 3D printing of composite calcium phosphate and collagen scaffolds for bone regeneration. *Biomaterials*, (2014), 35, 4026–4034.

471. Tamimi F., Kumarasami B., Doillon C., Gbureck U., Nihouannen D.L., Cabarcos E.L., Barralet J.E., Brushite-collagen composites for bone regeneration. *Acta Biomater.*, (2008), 4, 1315–1321.

472. Mai R., Reinstorf A., Pilling E., Hlawitschka M., Jung R., Gelinsky M., Schneider M., Loukota R., Pompe W., Eckelt U., Stadlinger B., Histologic study of incorporation and resorption of a bone cement-collagen composite: an *in vivo* study in the minipig. *Oral Surg. Oral Med. Oral Pathol. Oral Radiol. Endod.*, (2008), 105, e9–e14.

473. Moreau J.L., Weir M.D., Xu H.H.K., Self-setting collagen-calcium phosphate bone cement: mechanical and cellular properties. *J. Biomed. Mater. Res. A*, (2009), 91A, 605–613.

474. Liu X., Wang X.M., Chen Z., Cui F.Z., Liu H.Y., Mao K., Wang Y., Injectable bone cement based on mineralized collagen. *J. Biomed. Mater. Res. B Appl. Biomater.*, (2010), 94B, 72–79.

475. Otsuka M., Nakagawa H., Ito A., Higuchi W.I., Effect of geometrical structure on drug release rate of a three-dimensionally perforated porous apatite/collagen composite cement. *J. Pharm. Sci.*, (2010), 99, 286–292.

476. Cui F.Z., Li Y., G.e, J., Self-assembly of mineralized collagen composites. *Mater. Sci. Eng. R*, (2007), 57, 1–27.

477. Hirota K., Nishihara K., Tanaka H., Pressure sintering of apatite-collagen composite. *Biomed. Mater. Eng.*, (1993), 3, 147–151.

478. Zahn D., Hochrein O., Kawska A., Brickmann J., Kniep R., Towards an atomistic understanding of apatite-collagen biomaterials: linking molecular simulation studies of complex-, crystal- and composite-formation to experimental findings. *J. Mater. Sci.*, (2007), 42, 8966–8973.

479. Silva C.C., Pinheiro A.G., Figueiro S.D., Goes J.C., Sasaki J.M., Miranda M.A.R., Sombra A.S.B., Piezoelectric properties of collagen-nanocrystalline hydroxyapatite composites. *J. Mater. Sci.*, (2002), 37, 2061–2070.

480. Yunoki S., Ikoma T., Tsuchiya A., Monkawa A., Ohta K., Sotome S., Shinomiya K., Tanaka J., Fabrication and mechanical and tissue ingrowth properties of unidirectionally porous hydroxyapatite/collagen composite. *J. Biomed. Mater. Res. B Appl. Biomater.*, (2007), 80B, 166–173.

481. Keeney M., Collin E., Pandit A., Multi-channelled collagen-calcium phosphate scaffolds: their physical properties and human cell response. *Tissue Eng. C*, (2009), 15, 265–273.

482. Chapman M.W., Bucholz R., Cornell C., Treatment of acute fractures with a collagen-calcium phosphate graft material: a randomized clinical trial. *J. Bone Joint Surg. (Am.)*, (1997), 79A, 495–502.

483. Rodrigues C.V.M., Serricella P., Linhares A.B.R., Guerdes R.M., Borojevic R., Rossi M.A., Duarte M.E.L., Farina M., Characterization of a bovine collagen-hydroxyapatite composite scaffold for bone tissue engineering. *Biomaterials*, (2003), 24, 4987–4997.

484. Miura K.-I., Anada T., Honda Y., Shiwaku Y., Kawai T., Echigo S., Takahashi T., Suzuki O., Characterization and bioactivity of nano-submicro octacalcium phosphate/gelatin composite. *Appl. Surf. Sci.*, (2013), 282, 138–145.

485. Kawai T., Echigo S., Matsui K., Tanuma Y., Takahashi T., Suzuki O., Kamakura S., First clinical application of octacalcium phosphate collagen composite in human bone defect. *Tissue Eng. A*, (2014), 20, 1336–1341.

486. Lickorish D., Ramshaw J.A.M., Werkmeister J.A., Glattauer V., Howlett C.R., Development of a collagen-hydroxyapatite composite biomaterial via biomimetic process. *J. Biomed. Mater. Res. A*, (2004), 68A, 19–27.

487. Sionkowska A., Kozłowska J., Characterization of collagen/hydroxy-apatite composite sponges as a potential bone substitute. *Int. J. Biol. Macromol.*, (2010), 47, 483–487.

488. Hsu F.Y., Chueh S.C., Wang J.Y., Microspheres of hydroxyapatite/reconstituted collagen as supports for osteoblast cell growth. *Biomaterials*, (1999), 20, 1931–1936.

489. Wu T.J., Huang H.H., Lan C.W., Lin C.H., Hsu F.Y., Wang Y.J., Studies on the microspheres comprised of reconstituted collagen and hydroxyapa-tite. *Biomaterials*, (2004), 25, 651–658.

490. Wei Q., Lu J., Wang Q., Fan H., Zhang X., Novel synthesis strategy for composite hydrogel of collagen/hydroxyapatite-microsphere originating from conversion of $CaCO_3$ templates. *Nanotechnology*, (2015), 26, 115605.

491. Liao S.S., Watari F., Uo M., Ohkawa S., Tamura K., Wang W., Cui F.Z., The preparation and characteristics of a carbonated hydroxyapatite/collagen composite at room temperature. *J. Biomed. Mater. Res. B Appl. Biomater.*, (2005), 74B, 817–821.

492. Yokoyama A., Gelinsky M., Kawasaki T., Kohgo T., König U., Pompe W., Watari F., Biomimetic porous scaffolds with high elasticity made from mineralized collagen – an animal study. *J. Biomed. Mater. Res. B Appl. Biomater.*, (2005), 75B, 464–472.

493. Zou C., Weng W., Deng X.J., Cheng K., Liu X., Du P., Shen G., Han G., Preparation and characterization of porous β-tricalcium phosphate/collagen composites with an integrated structure. *Biomaterials*, (2005), 26, 5276–5284.

494. Martins V.C.A., Goissis G., Nonstoichiometric hydroxyapatite-anionic collagen composite as a support for the double sustained release of gentamicin and norfloxacin/ciprofloxacin. *Artif. Organs*, (2000), 24, 224–230.

495. Gotterbarm T., Richter W., Jung M., Berardi-Vilei S., Mainil-Varlet P., Yamashita T., Breusch S.J., An *in vivo* study of a growth-factor enhanced, cell free, two-layered collagen-tricalcium phosphate in deep osteochondral defects. *Biomaterials*, (2006), 27, 3387–3395.

496. Martins V.C., Goissis G., Ribeiro A.C., Marcantonio E., Jr., Bet M.R., The controlled release of antibiotic by hydroxyapatite: anionic collagen composites. *Artif. Organs*, (1998), 22, 215–221.

497. Jayaraman M., Subramanian M.V., Preparation and characterization of two new composites: collagen-brushite and collagen-octacalcium phosphate. *Medical Sci. Monitor*, (2002), 8, BR481–BR487.

498. Matsui K., Matsui A., Handa T., Kawai T., Suzuki O., Kamakura S., Echigo S., Bone regeneration by octacalcium phosphate collagen composites in a dog alveolar cleft model. *Int. J. Oral Maxillofac. Surg.*, (2010), 39, 1218–1225.

499. Iibuchi S., Matsui K., Kawai T., Sasaki K., Suzuki O., Kamakura S., Echigo S., Octacalcium phosphate (OCP) collagen composites enhance bone healing in a dog tooth extraction socket model. *Int. J. Oral Maxillofac. Surg.*, (2010), 39, 161–168.

500. Kawai T., Matsui K., Ezoe Y., Kajii F., Suzuki O., Takahashi T., Kamakura S., Efficacy of octacalcium phosphate collagen composite for titanium dental implants in dogs. *Materials*, (2018), 11, 229.

501. Xia Z., Wei M., Biomimetic fabrication of collagen-apatite scaffolds for bone tissue regeneration. *J. Biomater. Tissue Eng.*, (2013), 3, 369–384.

502. Ikeda H., Yamaza T., Yoshinari M., Ohsaki Y., Ayukawa Y., Kido M.A., Inoue T., Shimono M., Koyano K., Tanaka T., Ultrastructural and immunoelectron microscopic studies of the peri-implant epithelium-implant (Ti-6Al-4V) interface of rat maxilla. *J. Periodontol.*, (2000), 71, 961–973.

503. Uchida M., Oyane A., Kim H.M., Kokubo T., Ito A., Biomimetic coating of laminin-apatite composite on titanium metal and its excellent cell-adhesive properties. *Adv. Mater.*, (2004), 16, 1071–1074.

504. Oyane A., Uchida M., Ito A., Laminin-apatite composite coating to enhance cell adhesion to ethylene-vinyl alcohol copolymer. *J. Biomed. Mater. Res. A*, (2005), 72A, 168–174.

505. Oyane A., Uchida M., Onuma K., Ito A., Spontaneous growth of a laminin-apatite nano-composite in a metastable calcium phosphate solution. *Biomaterials*, (2006), 27, 167–175.

506. Oyane A., Tsurushima H., Ito A., Highly efficient gene transfer system using a laminin-DNA-apatite composite layer. *J. Gene Med.*, (2010), 12, 194–206.

507. Oyane A., Wang X., Sogo Y., Ito A., Tsurushima H., Calcium phosphate composite layers for surface-mediated gene transfer. *Acta Biomater.*, (2012), 8, 2034–2046.

508. Yaylaoglu M.B., Korkusuz P., Ors U., Korkusuz F., Hasirci V., Development of a calcium phosphate-gelatin composite as a bone substitute and its use in drug release. *Biomaterials*, (1999), 20, 711–719.

509. Kim H.W., Knowles J.C., Kim H.E., Porous scaffolds of gelatin-hydroxyapatite nanocomposites obtained by biomimetic approach: characterization and antibiotic drug release. *J. Biomed. Mater. Res. B Appl. Biomater.*, (2005), 74B, 686–698.

510. Hillig W.B., Choi Y., Murtha S., Natravali N., Ajayan P., An open-pored gelatin/hydroxyapatite composite as a potential bone substitute. *J. Mater. Sci. Mater. Med.*, (2008), 19, 11–17.

511. Chang M.C., Douglas W.H., Tanaka J., Organic-inorganic interaction and the growth mechanism of hydroxyapatite crystals in gelatin matrices between 37 and 80 °C. *J. Mater. Sci. Mater. Med.*, (2006), 17, 387–396.

512. Chang M.C., Douglas W.H., Cross-linkage of hydroxyapatite/gelatin nanocomposite using imide-based zero-length cross-linker. *J. Mater. Sci. Mater. Med.*, (2007), 18, 2045–2051.

513. Liu X., Smith L.A., Hu J., Ma P.X., Biomimetic nanofibrous gelatin/apatite composite scaffolds for bone tissue engineering. *Biomaterials*, (2009), 30, 2252–2258.

514. Lin H.R., Yeh Y.J., Porous alginate/hydroxyapatite composite scaffolds for bone tissue engineering: preparation, characterization and *in vitro* studies. *J. Biomed. Mater. Res. B Appl. Biomater.*, (2004), 71B, 52–65.

515. Turco G., Marsich E., Bellomo F., Semeraro S., Donati I., Brun F., Grandolfo M., Accardo A., Paoletti S., Alginate/hydroxyapatite biocomposite for bone ingrowth: a trabecular structure with high and isotropic connectivity. *Biomacromolecules*, (2009), 10, 1575–1583.

516. Chae T., Yang H., Leung V., Ko F., Troczynski T., Novel biomimetic hydroxyapatite/alginate nanocomposite fibrous scaffolds for bone tissue regeneration. *J. Mater. Sci. Mater. Med.*, (2013), 24, 1885–1894.

517. Cuozzo R.C., da Leão, M.H.M.R., de Gobbo L.A., da Rocha D.N., Ayad N.M.E., Trindade W., Costa A.M., da Silva M.H.P., Zinc alginate-hydroxyapatite composite microspheres for bone repair. *Ceram. Int.*, (2014), 40, 11369–11375.

518. Li S., Kan B., Zhao K., Ren T., Lin B., Wei J., Chen T., Preparation of tricalcium phosphate-calcium alginate composite flat sheet membranes and their application for protein release. *Polym. Compos.*, (2015), 36, 1899–1906.

519. Won J.E., El-Fiqi A., Jegal S.H., Han C.M., Lee E.J., Knowles J.C., Kim H.W., Gelatin-apatite bone mimetic co-precipitates incorporated within biopolymer matrix to improve mechanical and biological properties useful for hard tissue repair. *J. Biomater. Appl.*, (2014), 28, 1213–1225.

520. Sarkar C., Kumari P., Anuvrat K., Sahu S.K., Chakraborty J., Garai S., Synthesis and characterization of mechanically strong carboxymethyl cellulose–gelatin–hydroxyapatite nanocomposite for load-bearing orthopedic application. *J. Mater. Sci.*, (2018), 53, 230–246.

521. Yamaguchi I., Tokuchi K., Fukuzaki H., Koyama Y., Takakuda K., Monma H., Tanaka J., Preparation and microstructure analysis of chitosan/hydroxyapatite nanocomposites. *J. Biomed. Mater. Res.*, (2001), 55, 20–27.

522. Zhang Y., Ni M., Zhang M.Q., Ratner B., Calcium phosphate – chitosan composite scaffolds for bone tissue engineering. *Tissue Eng.*, (2003), 9, 337–345.

523. Tang X.J., Gui L., Lü, X.Y., Hard tissue compatibility of natural hydroxyapatite/chitosan composite. *Biomed. Mater.*, (2008), 3, 044115.

524. Zhang Y., Venugopal J.R., El-Turki A., Ramakrishna S., Su B., Lim C.T., Electrospun biomimetic nanocomposite nanofibers of hydroxyapatite/chitosan for bone tissue engineering. *Biomaterials*, (2008), 29, 4314–4322.

525. Cai X., Tong H., Shen X., Chen W., Yan J., Hu J., Preparation and characterization of homogeneous chitosan-polylactic acid/hydroxyapatite nanocomposite for bone tissue engineering and evaluation of its mechanical properties. *Acta Biomater.*, (2010), 5, 2693–2703.

526. Ge H., Zhao B., Lai Y., Hu X., Zhang D., Hu K., From crabshell to chitosan-hydroxyapatite composite material via a biomorphic mineralization synthesis method. *J. Mater. Sci. Mater. Med.*, (2010), 21, 1781–1787.

527. Onoki T., Nakahira A., Tago T., Hasegawa Y., Kuno T., Novel low temperature processing techniques for apatite ceramics and chitosan polymer composite bulk materials and its mechanical properties. *Appl. Surf. Sci.*, (2012), 262, 263–266.

528. Zugravu M.V., Smith R.A., Reves B.T., Jennings J.A., Cooper J.O., Haggard W.O., Bumgardner J.D., Physical properties and *in vitro* evaluation of collagen-chitosan-calcium phosphate microparticle-based scaffolds for bone tissue regeneration. *J. Biomater. Appl.*, (2013), 28, 566–579.

529. Fernández T., Olave G., Valencia C.H., Arce S., Quinn J.M.W., Thouas G.A., Chen Q.Z., Effects of calcium phosphate/chitosan composite on bone healing in rats: calcium phosphate induces osteon formation. *Tissue Eng. A*, (2014), 20, 1948–1960.

530. Tang S., Tian B., Guo Y.J., Zhu Z.A., Guo Y.P., Chitosan/carbonated hydroxyapatite composite coatings: fabrication, structure and biocompatibility. *Surf. Coat. Technol.*, (2014), 251, 210–216.

531. Kucharska M., Walenko K., Lewandowska-Szumieł, M., Brynk T., Jaroszewicz J., Ciach T., Chitosan and composite microsphere-based scaffold for bone tissue engineering: evaluation of tricalcium phosphate content influence on physical and biological properties. *J. Mater. Sci. Mater. Med.*, (2015), 26, 143 (12 pages).

532. Park K.H., Kim S.J., Hwang M.J., Song H.J., Park Y.J., Biomimetic fabrication of calcium phosphate/chitosan nanohybrid composite in modified simulated body fluids. *Express Polym. Lett.*, (2017), 11, 14–20.

533. Wan A.C.A., Khor E., Hastings G.W., Preparation of a chitin-apatite composite by *in situ* precipitation onto porous chitin scaffolds. *J. Biomed. Mater. Res.*, (1998), 41, 541–548.

534. Wan A.C.A., Khor E., Hastings G.W., Hydroxyapatite modified chitin as potential hard tissue substitute material. *J. Biomed. Mater. Res.*, (1997), 38, 235–241.

535. Geçer A., Yldz N., Erol M., Çalml A., Synthesis of chitin calcium phosphate composite in different growth media. *Polym. Composite*, (2008), 29, 84–91.

536. Dong H., Ye J.D., Wang X.P., Yang J.J., Preparation of calcium phosphate cement tissue engineering scaffold reinforced with chitin fiber. *J. Inorg. Mater.*, (2007), 22, 1007–1010.

537. Silva S.S., Duarte A.R.C., Oliveira J.M., Mano J.F., Reis R.L., Alternative methodology for chitin–hydroxyapatite composites using ionic liquids and supercritical fluid technology. *J. Bioact. Compat. Polym.*, (2013), 28, 481–491.

538. Wang J., Sun Q.Z., Gao J., Liu D.M., Meng X.C., Li M.Q., Preparation and properties on silk fibers reinforced hydroxyapatite/chitosan composites. *Adv. Mater. Res.*, (2010), 105–106, 557–560.

539. Zhang Y., Reddy V.J., Wong S.Y., Li X., Su B., Ramakrishna S., Lim C.T., Enhanced biomineralization in osteoblasts on a novel electrospun biocomposite nanofibrous substrate of hydroxyapatite/collagen/chitosan. *Tissue Eng. A*, (2010), 16, 1949–1960.

540. Kousalya G.N., Gandhi R.M., Sundaram S.C., Meenakshi S., Synthesis of nano-hydroxyapatite chitin/chitosan hybrid biocomposites for the removal of Fe(III). *Carbohydr. Polym.*, (2010), 82, 594–599.

541. Sundaram C.S., Viswanathan N., Meenakshi S., Uptake of fluoride by nano-hydroxyapatite/chitosan, a bioinorganic composite. *Bioresour. Technol.*, (2008), 99, 8226–8230.

542. Sundaram C.S., Viswanathan N., Meenakshi S., Fluoride sorption by nano-hydroxyapatite/chitin composite. *J. Hazard. Mater.*, (2009), 172, 147–151.

543. Wen H.B., de Wijn J.R., van Blitterswijk C.A., de Groot K., Incorporation of bovine serum albumin in calcium phosphate coating on titanium. *J. Biomed. Mater. Res.*, (1999), 46, 245–252.

544. Liu T.Y., Chen S.Y., Liu D.M., Liou S.C., On the study of BSA-loaded calcium-deficient hydroxyapatite nano-carriers for controlled drug delivery. *J. Control. Release*, (2005), 107, 112–121.

545. Liu Y., Hunziker E., Randall N., de Groot K., Layrolle P., Proteins incorporated into biomimetically prepared calcium phosphate coatings modulate their mechanical strength and dissolution rate. *Biomaterials*, (2003), 24, 65–70.

546. Dorozhkin S.V., Dorozhkina E.I., The influence of bovine serum albumin on the crystallization of calcium phosphates from a revised simulated body fluid. *Colloid Surface A*, (2003), 215, 191–199.

547. Fu H.H., Hu Y.H., McNelis T., Hollinger J.O., A calcium phosphate-based gene delivery system. *J. Biomed. Mater. Res. A*, (2005), 74A, 40–48.

548. Bisht S., Bhakta G., Mitra S., Maitra A., pDNA loaded calcium phosphate nanoparticles: highly efficient non-viral vector for gene delivery. *Int. J. Pharm.*, (2005), 288, 157–168.

549. Kakizawa Y., Miyata K., Furukawa S., Kataoka K., Size-controlled formation of a calcium phosphate-based organic-inorganic hybrid vector for gene delivery using poly(ethylene glycol)-block-poly(aspartic acid). *Adv. Mater.*, (2004), 16, 699–702.

550. Singh R., Saxena A., Mozumdar S., Calcium phosphate – DNA nanocomposites: morphological studies and their bile duct infusion for liver-directed gene therapy. *Int. J. Appl. Ceram. Technol.*, (2008), 5, 1–10.

551. Oyane A., Araki H., Sogo Y., Ito A., Tsurushima H., Coprecipitation of DNA and calcium phosphate using an infusion fluid mixture. *Key Eng. Mater.*, (2013), 529–530, 465–470.

552. Sporysh I., Shynkaruk E., Lysko O., Shynkaruk A., Dubok V., Buzaneva E., Ritter U., Scharff P., Biomimetic hydroxyapatite nanocrystals in composites with C$_{60}$ and Au-DNA nanoparticles: IR-spectral study. *Mater. Sci. Eng. B*, (2010), 169, 128–133.

553. Taguchi T., Kishida A., Akashi M., Hydroxyapatite formation on/in poly(vinyl alcohol) hydrogel matrices using a novel alternate soaking process. *Chem. Lett.*, (1998), 8, 711–712.

554. Tachaboonyakiat W., Serizawa T., Akashi M., Hydroxyapatite formation on/in biodegradable chitosan hydrogels by an alternate soaking process. *Polym. J.*, (2001), 33, 177–181.

555. Schnepp Z.A.C., Gonzalez-McQuire R., Mann S., Hybrid biocomposites based on calcium phosphate mineralization of self-assembled supramolecular hydrogels. *Adv. Mater.*, (2006), 18, 1869–1872.

556. Patel M., Patel K.J., Caccamese J.F., Coletti D.P., Sauk J.J., Fisher J.P., Characterization of cyclic acetal hydroxyapatite nanocomposites for craniofacial tissue engineering. *J. Biomed. Mater. Res. A*, (2010), 94A, 408–418.

557. Bigi A., Boanini E., Gazzano M., Kojdecki M.A., Rubini K., Microstructural investigation of hydroxyapatite-polyelectrolyte composites. *J. Mater. Chem.*, (2004), 14, 274–279.

558. Bigi A., Boanini E., Gazzano M., Rubini K., Torricelli P., Nanocrystalline hydroxyapatite-polyaspartate composites. *Biomed. Mater. Eng.*, (2004), 14, 573–579.

559. Boanini E., Fini M., Gazzano M., Bigi A., Hydroxyapatite nanocrystals modified with acidic amino acids. *Eur. J. Inorg. Chem.*, (2006), 4821–4826, doi: 10.1002/ejic.200600423.

560. Boanini E., Torricelli P., Gazzano M., Giardino R., Bigi A., Nanocomposites of hydroxyapatite with aspartic acid and glutamic acid and their interaction with osteoblast-like cells. *Biomaterials*, (2006), 27, 4428–4433.

561. Sánchez-Salcedo S., Nieto A., Vallet-Regi M., Hydroxyapatite/β-tricalcium phosphate/agarose macroporous scaffolds for bone tissue engineering. *Chem. Eng. J.*, (2005), 137, 62–71.

562. Román, J., Cabañas M.V., Peña, J., Doadrio J.C., Vallet-Regi M., An optimized β-tricalcium phosphate and agarose scaffold fabrication technique. *J. Biomed. Mater. Res. A*, (2008), 84A, 99–107.

563. Alcaide M., Serrano M.C., Pagani R., Sánchez-Salcedo S., Nieto A., Vallet-Regí, M., Portolés, M.T., L929 fibroblast and SAOS-2 osteoblast response to hydroxyapatite-βTCP/ agarose biomaterial. *J. Biomed. Mater. Res. A*, (2009), 89A, 539–549.

564. Abiraman S., Varma H., Umashankar P., John A., Fibrin sealant as an osteoinductive protein in a mouse model. *Biomaterials*, (2002), 23, 3023–3031.

565. Wittkampf A., Fibrin sealant as sealant for hydroxyapatite granules. *J. Craniomaxillofac. Surg.*, (1989), 17, 179–181.

566. d'Arc M.B., Daculsi G., Micro macroporous biphasic ceramics and fibrin sealant as a mouldable material for bone reconstruction in chronic otitis media surgery: a 15 years experience. *J. Mater. Sci. Mater. Med.*, (2003), 14, 229–233.

567. le Nihouannen D., Guehennec L.L., Rouillon T., Pilet P., Bilban M., Layrolle P., Daculsi G., Micro-architecture of calcium phosphate granules and fibrin glue composites for bone tissue engineering. *Biomaterials*, (2006), 27, 2716–2722.

568. le Nihouannen D., Saffarzadeh A., Aguado E., Goyenvalle E., Gauthier O., Moreau F., Pilet P., Spaethe R., Daculsi G., Layrolle P., Osteogenic properties of calcium phosphate ceramics and fibrin glue based composites. *J. Mater. Sci. Mater. Med.*, (2007), 18, 225–235.

569. le Nihouannen D., Goyenvalle E., Aguado E., Pilet P., Bilban M., Daculsi G., Layrolle P., Hybrid composites of calcium phosphate granules, fibrin glue, and bone marrow for skeletal repair. *J. Biomed. Mater. Res. A*, (2007), 81A, 399–408.

570. Yoh R., Matsumoto T., Sasaki J.I., Sohmura T., Biomimetic fabrication of fibrin/apatite composite material. *J. Biomed. Mater. Res. A*, (2008), 87A, 222–228.

571. Cui G., Li J., Lei W., Bi L., Tang P., Liang Y., Tao S., Wang Y., The mechanical and biological properties of an injectable calcium phosphate cement-fibrin glue composite for bone regeneration. *J. Biomed. Mater. Res. B Appl. Biomater.*, (2010), 92B, 377–385.

572. Boanini E., Torricelli P., Gazzano M., Giardino R., Bigi A., Alendronate-hydroxyapatite nanocomposites and their interaction with osteoclasts and osteoblast-like cells. *Biomaterials*, (2008), 29, 790–796.

573. Wang L., Nemoto R., Senna M., Microstructure and chemical states of hydroxyapatite/silk fibroin nanocomposites synthesized via a wet-mechanochemical route. *J. Nanopart. Res.*, (2002), 4, 535–540.

574. Nemoto R., Wang L., Ikoma T., Tanaka J., Senna M., Preferential alignment of hydroxyapatite crystallites in nanocomposites with chemically disintegrated silk fibroin. *J. Nanopart. Res.*, (2004), 6, 259–265.

575. Wang L., Li C.Z., Senna M., High-affinity integration of hydroxyapatite nanoparticles with chemically modified silk fibroin. *J. Nanopart. Res.*, (2007), 9, 919–929.

576. Li L., Wei K.M., Lin F., Kong X.D., Yao J.M., Effect of silicon on the formation of silk fibroin/calcium phosphate composite. *J. Mater. Sci. Mater. Med.*, (2008), 19, 577–582.

577. Fan C., Li J., Xu G., He H., Ye X., Chen Y., Sheng X., Fu J., He D., Facile fabrication of nano-hydroxyapatite/silk fibroin composite via a simplified coprecipitation route. *J. Mater. Sci.*, (2010), 45, 5814–5819.

578. Liu H., Xu G.W., Wang Y.F., Zhao H.S., Xiong S., Wu Y., Heng B.C., An C.R., Zhu G.H., Xie D.H., Composite scaffolds of nano-hydroxyapatite and silk fibroin enhance mesenchymal stem cell-based bone regeneration via the interleukin 1 alpha autocrine/paracrine signaling loop. *Biomaterials*, (2015), 49, 103–112.

579. Farokhi M., Mottaghitalab F., Samani S., Shokrgozar M.A., Kundu S.C., Reis R.L., Fatahi Y., Kaplan D.L., Silk fibroin/hydroxyapatite composites for bone tissue engineering. *Biotechnol. Adv.*, (2018), 36, 68–91.

580. Farokhi M., Mottaghitalab F., Samani S., Shokrgozar M.A., Kundu S.C., Reis R.L., Fatahi Y., Kaplan D.L., Silk fibroin/hydroxyapatite composites for bone tissue engineering. *Biotechnol. Adv.*, (2018), 36, 68–91.

581. Salama A., Neumann M., Günter C., Taubert A., Ionic liquid-assisted formation of cellulose/calcium phosphate hybrid materials. *Beilstein J. Nanotechnol.*, (2014), 5, 1553–1568.

582. Wang L., Li C.Z., Preparation and physicochemical properties of a novel hydroxyapatite/chitosan-silk fibroin composite. *Carbohydr. Polym.*, (2007), 68, 740–745.

583. Shahbazarab Z., Teimouri A., Chermahini A.N., Azadi M., Fabrication and characterization of nanobiocomposite scaffold of zein/chitosan/ nanohydroxyapatite prepared by freeze-drying method for bone tissue engineering. *Int. J. Biol. Macromol.*, (2018), 108, 1017–1027.

584. Oliveira J.M., Costa S.A., Leonor I.B., Malafaya P.B., Mano J.F., Reis R.L., Novel hydroxyapatite/carboxymethylchitosan composite scaffolds prepared through an innovative "autocatalytic" electroless coprecipitation route. *J. Biomed. Mater. Res. A*, (2009), 88, 470–480.

585. Sogo Y., Ito A., Matsuno T., Oyane A., Tamazawa G., Satoh T., Yamazaki A., Uchimura E., Ohno T., Fibronectin-calcium phosphate composite layer on hydroxyapatite to enhance adhesion., cell spread and osteogenic differentiation of human mesenchymal stem cells *in vitro*. *Biomed. Mater.*, (2007), 2, 116–123.

586. Rhee S.H., Suetsugu Y., Tanaka J., Biomimetic configurational arrays of hydroxyapatite nanocrystals on bio-organics. *Biomaterials*, (2001), 22, 2843–2847.

587. Cross K.J., Huq N.L., Palamara J.E., Perich J.W., Reynolds E.C., Physicochemical characterization of casein phosphopeptide-amorphous calcium phosphate nanocomplexes. *J. Biol. Chem.*, (2005), 280, 15362–15369.

588. Dimopoulou M., Ritzoulis C., Papastergiadis E.S., Panayiotou C., Composite materials based on okra hydrocolloids and hydroxyapatite. *Food Hydrocolloid*, (2014), 42, 348–354.

589. Nakata R., Tachibana A., Tanabe T., Preparation of keratin hydrogel/ hydroxyapatite composite and its evaluation as a controlled drug release carrier. *Mater. Sci. Eng. C*, (2014), 41, 59–64.

590. Manda M.G., da Silva L.P., Cerqueira M.T., Pereira D.R., Oliveira M.B., Mano J.F., Marques A.P., Oliveira J.M., Correlo V.M., Reis R.L., Gellan gum-hydroxyapatite composite spongy-like hydrogels for bone tissue engineering. *J. Biomed. Mater. Res. A*, (2018), 106A, 479–490.

591. Yu P., Bao R.Y., Shi X.J., Yang W., Yang M.B., Self-assembled high-strength hydroxyapatite/graphene oxide/chitosan composite hydrogel for bone tissue engineering. *Carbohyd. Polym.*, (2017), 155, 507–515.

592. Li C., Born A.K., Schweizer T., Zenobi-Wong M., Cerruti M., Mezzenga R., Amyloid-hydroxyapatite bone biomimetic composites. *Adv. Mater.*, (2014), 26, 3207–3212.

593. Kolanthai E., Colon V.S.D., Sindu P.A., Chandra V.S., Karthikeyan K.R., Babu M.S., Sundaram S.M., Palanichamy M., Kalkura S.N., Effect of solvent; enhancing the wettability and engineering the porous structure of a calcium phosphate/agarose composite for drug delivery. *RSC Adv.*, (2015), 5, 18301–18311.

594. Krukowski S., Lysenko N., Kolodziejski W., Synthesis and characterization of nanocrystalline composites containing calcium hydroxyapatite and glycine. *J. Solid State Chem.*, (2018), 264, 59–67.

595. Jung J.Y., Hong Y.J., Choi Y.S., Jeong S., Lee W.K., A new method for the preparation of bioactive calcium phosphate films hybridized with 1α,25-dihydroxyvitamin D₃. *J. Mater. Sci. Mater. Med.*, (2010), 20, 2441–2453.

596. Killion J.A., Geever L.M., Devine D.M., Higginbotham C.L., Fabrication and *in vitro* biological evaluation of photopolymerisable hydroxyapatite hydrogel composites for bone regeneration. *J. Biomater. Appl.*, (2014), 28, 1274–1283.

597. Shchukin D.G., Sukhorukov G.B., Möhwald H., Biomimetic fabrication of nanoengineered hydroxyapatite/polyelectrolyte composite shell. *Chem. Mater.*, (2003), 15, 3947–3950.

598. Busch S., Dolhaine H., DuChesne A., Heinz S., Hochrein O., Laeri F., Podebrad O., Vietze U., Weiland T., Kniep R., Biomimetic morphogenesis of fluorapatite-gelatin composites: fractal growth, the question

of intrinsic electric fields, core/shell assemblies, hollow spheres and reorganization of denatured collagen. *Eur. J. Inorg. Chem.*, (1999), 1999, 1643–1653.

599. Simon P., Schwarz U., Kniep R., Hierarchical architecture and real structure in a biomimetic nano-composite of fluorapatite with gelatine: a model system for steps in dentino- and osteogenesis? *J. Mater. Chem.*, (2005), 15, 4992–4996.

600. Tlatlik H., Simon P., Kawska A., Zahn D., Kniep R., Biomimetic fluorapatite-gelatin nanocomposites: pre-structuring of gelatin matrices by ion impregnation and its effect on form development. *Angew. Chem. Int. Ed. Engl.*, (2006), 45, 1905–1910.

601. Simon P., Zahn D., Lichte H., Kniep R., Intrinsic electric dipole fields and the induction of hierarchical form developments in fluorapatite-gelatin nanocomposites: a general principle for morphogenesis of biominerals? *Angew. Chem. Int. Ed. Engl.*, (2006), 45, 1911–1915.

602. Kniep R., Simon P., "Hidden" hierarchy of microfibrils within 3D-periodic fluorapatite-gelatin nanocomposites: development of complexity and form in a biomimetic system. *Angew. Chem. Int. Ed. Engl.*, (2008), 47, 1405–1409.

603. Brickmann J., Paparcone R., Kokolakis S., Zahn D., Duchstein P., Carrillocabrera W., Simon P., Kniep R., Fluorapatite-gelatine nanocomposite superstructures: new insights into a biomimetic system of high complexity. *ChemPhysChem*, (2010), 11, 1851–1853.

604. Vyalikh A., Simon P., Rosseeva E., Buder J., Kniep R., Scheler U., Intergrowth and interfacial structure of biomimetic fluorapatite-gelatin nanocomposite: a solid-state NMR study. *J. Phys. Chem. B*, (2014), 118, 724–730.

605. Gashti M.P., Stir M., Hulliger J., Synthesis of bone-like micro-porous calcium phosphate/iota-carrageenan composites by gel diffusion. *Colloid Surface B*, (2013), 110, 426–433.

606. Jacoveila P.F., Use of calcium hydroxylapatite (Radiesse®) for facial augmentation. *Clin. Interv. Aging*, (2008), 3, 161–174.

607. Lizzul P.F., Narurkar V.A., The role of calcium hydroxylapatite (Radiesse®) in nonsurgical aesthetic rejuvenation. *J. Drugs Dermatol.*, (2010), 9, 446–450.

608. Klesing J., Chernousova S., Kovtun A., Neumann S., Ruiz L., Gonzalez-Calbet J.M., Vallet-Regi M., Heumann R., Epple M., An injectable paste of calcium phosphate nanorods, functionalized with nucleic acids, for cell transfection and gene silencing. *J. Mater. Chem.*, (2010), 20, 6144–6148.

609. Thai V.V., Lee B.T., Fabrication of calcium phosphate-calcium sulfate injectable bone substitute using hydroxy-propyl-methyl-cellulose and citric acid. *J. Mater. Sci. Mater. Med.*, (2010), 21, 1867–1874.

610. Low K.L., Tan S.H., Zein S.H.S., Roether J.A., Mouriño, V., Boccaccini A.R., Calcium phosphate-based composites as injectable bone substitute materials. *J. Biomed. Mater. Res. B Appl. Biomater.*, (2010), 94B, 273–286.

611. D'Este M., Eglin D., Hydrogels in calcium phosphate moldable and injectable bone substitutes: sticky excipients or advanced 3-D carriers? *Acta Biomater.*, (2013), 9, 5421–5430.

612. Weiss P., Gauthier O., Bouler J.M., Grimandi G., Daculsi G., Injectable bone substitute using a hydrophilic polymer. *Bone*, (1999), 25(2), 67S–70S.

613. Daculsi G., Weiss P., Bouler J.M., Gauthier O., Millot F., Aguado E., Biphasic calcium phosphate/hydrosoluble polymer composites: a new concept for bone and dental substitution biomaterials. *Bone*, (1999), 25(2), 59S–61S.

614. Turczyn R., Weiss P., Lapkowski M., Daculsi G., *In situ* self-hardening bioactive composite for bone and dental surgery. *J. Biomater. Sci. Polym. Edn.*, (2000), 11, 217–223.

615. Bennett S., Connolly K., Lee D.R., Jiang Y., Buck D., Hollinger J.O., Gruskin E.A., Initial biocompatibility studies of a novel degradable polymeric bone substitute that hardens *in situ*. *Bone*, (1996), 19, 101S–107S.

616. Bongio M., van den Beucken J.J.J.P., Nejadnik M.R., Leeuwenburgh S.C.G., Kinard L.A., Kasper F.K., Mikos A.G., Jansen J.A., Biomimetic modification of synthetic hydrogels by incorporation of adhesive peptides and calcium phosphate nanoparticles: *in vitro* evaluation of cell behavior. *Eur. Cell. Mater.*, (2011), 22, 359–376.

617. Bongio M., van den Beucken J.J.J.P., Nejadnik M.R., Birgani Z.T., Habibovic P., Kinard L.A., Kasper F.K., Mikos A.G., Leeuwenburgh S.C.G., Jansen J.A., Subcutaneous tissue response and osteogenic performance of calcium phosphate nanoparticle-enriched hydrogels in the tibial medullary cavity of guinea pigs. *Acta Biomater.*, (2013), 9, 5464–5474.

618. Chernousova S., Klesing J., Soklakova N., Epple M., A genetically active nano-calcium phosphate paste for bone substitution, encoding the formation of BMP-7 and VEGF-A. *RSC Adv.*, (2013), 3, 11155–11161.

619. Yu B., Zhang Y., Li X., Wang Q., Ouyang Y., Xia Y., Lin B., Li S., Fan Y., Chen Y., The use of injectable chitosan/nanohydroxyapatite/collagen composites with bone marrow mesenchymal stem cells to promote ectopic bone formation *in vivo*. *J. Nanomater.*, (2013), 2013, 506593.

620. Bodakhe S., Verma S., Garkhal K., Samal S.K., Sharma S.S., Kumar N., Injectable photocrosslinkable nanocomposite based on poly(glycerol sebacate) fumarate and hydroxyapatite: development, biocompatibility and bone regeneration in a rat calvarial bone defect model. *Nanomedicine*, (2013), 8, 1777–1795.

621. Fricain J.C., Aid R., Lanouar S., Maurel D.B., le Nihouannen D., Delmond S., Letourneur D., Vilamitjana J.A., Catros S., *In-vitro* and *in-vivo* design and validation of an injectable polysaccharide-hydroxyapatite composite material for sinus floor augmentation. *Dent. Mater.*, (2018), 34, 1024–1035.

622. Lin G., Cosimbescu L., Karin N.J., Tarasevich B.J., Injectable and thermosensitive PLGA-g-PEG hydrogels containing hydroxyapatite: preparation, characterization and *in vitro* release behavior. *Biomed. Mater.*, (2012), 7, 024107.

623. Nejadnik M.R., Yang X., Bongio M., Alghamdi H.S., van den Beucken J.J.J.P., Huysmans M.C., Jansen J.A., Hilborn J., Ossipov D., Leeuwenburgh S.C.G., Self-healing hybrid nanocomposites consisting of bisphosphonated hyaluronan and calcium phosphate nanoparticles. *Biomaterials*, (2014), 35, 6918–6929.

624. Munarin F., Petrini P., Gentilini R., Pillai R.S., Dirè, S., Tanzi M.C., Sglavo V.M., Micro- and nano-hydroxyapatite as active reinforcement for soft biocomposites. *Int. J. Biol. Macromol.*, (2015), 72, 199–209.

625. Douglas T.E.L., Schietse J., Zima A., Gorodzha S., Parakhonskiy B.V., Khalenkow D., Shkarin R., Ivanova A., Baumbach T., Weinhardt V., Stevens C.V., Vanhoorne V., Vervaet C., Balcaen L., Vanhaecke F., Ślósarczyk A., Surmeneva M.A., Surmenev R.A., Skirtach A.G., Novel self-gelling injectable hydrogel/alpha-tricalcium phosphate composites for bone regeneration: physiochemical and microcomputer tomographical characterization. *J. Biomed. Mater. Res. A*, (2018), 106A, 822–828.

626. Daculsi G., Rohanizadeh R., Weiss P., Bouler J.M., Crystal polymer interaction with new injectable bone substitute: SEM and HrTEM study. *J. Biomed. Mater. Res.*, (2000), 50, 1–7.

627. Grimande G., Weiss P., Millot F., Daculsi G., *In vitro* evaluation of a new injectable calcium phosphate material. *J. Biomed. Mater. Res.*, (1998), 39, 660–666.

628. Weiss P., Lapkowski M., LeGeros R.Z., Bouler J.M., Jean A., Daculsi G., FTIR spectroscopic study of an organic/mineral composite for bone and dental substitute materials. *J. Mater. Sci. Mater. Med.*, (1997), 8, 621–629.

629. Weiss P., Bohic S., Lapkowski M., Daculsi G., Application of FTIR microspectroscopy to the study of an injectable composite for bone and dental surgery. *J. Biomed. Mater. Res.*, (1998), 41, 167–170.

630. Schmitt M., Weiss P., Bourges X., del Valle G.A., Daculsi G., Crystallization at the polymer/calcium-phosphate interface in a sterilized injectable bone substitute IBS. *Biomaterials*, (2002), 23, 2789–2794.

631. Gauthier O., Müller R., von Stechow D., Lamy B., Weiss P., Bouler J.M., Aguado E., Daculsi G., *In vivo* bone regeneration with injectable calcium phosphate biomaterial: a three-dimensional micro-computed tomographic, biomechanical and SEM study. *Biomaterials*, (2005), 26, 5444–5453.

632. Weiss P., Layrolle P., Clergeau L.P., Enckel B., Pilet P., Amouriq Y., Daculsi G., Giumelli B., The safety and efficacy of an injectable bone substitute in dental sockets demonstrated in a human clinical trial. *Biomaterials*, (2007), 28, 3295–3305.

633. Fatimi A., Tassin J.F., Axelos M.A.V., Weiss P., The stability mechanisms of an injectable calcium phosphate ceramic suspension. *J. Mater. Sci. Mater. Med.*, (2010), 21, 1799–1809.

634. Trojani C., Boukhechba F., Scimeca J.C., Vandenbos F., Michiels J.F., Daculsi G., Boileau P., Weiss P., Carle G.F., Rochet N., Ectopic bone formation using an injectable biphasic calcium phosphate/Si-HPMC hydrogel composite loaded with undifferentiated bone marrow stromal cells. *Biomaterials*, (2006), 27, 3256–3264.

635. Zhang S.M., Lü, G., Clinical application of compound injectable bone substitutes in bone injury repair. *J. Clin. Rehabil. Tissue Eng. Res.*, (2009), 13, 10117–10120.

636. Daculsi G., Uzel P.A., Bourgeois N., le François T., Rouvillain J.L., Bourges X., Baroth S., New injectable bone substitute using reversible thermosensitive hydrogel and BCP granules: *in vivo* rabbit experiments. *Key Eng. Mater.*, (2009), 396–398, 457–460.

637. Iooss P., le Ray A.M., Grimandi G., Daculsi G., Merle C., A new injectable bone substitute combining poly(ε-caprolactone) microparticles with biphasic calcium phosphate granules. *Biomaterials*, (2001), 22, 2785–2794.

638. Bohner M., Design of ceramic-based cements and putties for bone graft substitution. *Eur. Cell Mater.*, (2010), 20, 1–12.

639. Wypych G., *Handbook of Fillers*, 3rd edn, ChemTec Publishing: New York, 2009, p. 800.

640. Almora-Barrios N., de Leeuw N.H., A density functional theory study of the interaction of collagen peptides with hydroxyapatite surfaces. *Langmuir*, (2010), 26, 14535–14542.

641. Zhang H.P., Lu X., Leng Y., Fang L., Qu S., Feng B., Weng J., Wang J., Molecular dynamics simulations on the interaction between polymers and hydroxyapatite with and without coupling agents. *Acta Biomater.*, (2009), 5, 1169–1181.

642. Rhee S.H., Lee J.D., Tanaka J., Nucleation of hydroxyapatite crystal through chemical interaction with collagen. *J. Am. Ceram. Soc.*, (2000), 83, 2890–2892.

643. Lin X., Li X., Fan H., Wen X., Lu J., Zhang X., *In situ* synthesis of bone-like apatite/collagen nano-composite at low temperature. *Mater. Lett.*, (2004), 58, 3569–3572.

644. Zhang W., Liao S.S., Cui F.Z., Hierarchical self-assembly of nanofibrils in mineralized collagen. *Chem. Mater.*, (2003), 15, 3221–3226.

645. Liu Q., de Wijn J.R., van Blitterswijk C.A., Covalent bonding of PMMA, PBMA and poly(HEMA) to hydroxyapatite particles. *J. Biomed. Mater. Res.*, (1998), 40, 257–263.

646. Li J., Chen Y.P., Yin Y., Yao F., Yao K., Modulation of nano-hydroxyapatite size via formation on chitosan-gelatin network film *in situ*. *Biomaterials*, (2007), 28, 781–790.

647. Zhou S., Zheng X., Yu X., Wang J., Weng J., Li X., Feng B., Yin M., Hydrogen bonding interaction of poly(D,L-lactide)/hydroxyapatite nanocomposites. *Chem. Mater.*, (2007), 19, 247–253.

648. Ficai A., Andronescu E., Ghitulica C., Voicu G., Trandafir V., Manzu D., Ficai M., Pall S., Colagen/hydroxyapatite interactions in composite biomaterials. *Materiale Plastice*, (2009), 46, 11–15.

649. Li J., Dou Y., Yang J., Yin Y., Zhang H., Yao F., Wang H., Yao K., Surface characterization and biocompatibility of micro- and nanohydroxyapatite/chitosan-gelatin network films. *Mater. Sci. Eng. C*, (2009), 29, 1207–1215.

650. Danilchenko S.N., Kalinkevich O.V., Kuznetsov V.N., Kalinkevich A.N., Kalinichenko T.G., Poddubny I.N., Starikov V.V., Sklyar A.M., Sukhodub L.F., Thermal transformations of the mineral component of composite biomaterials based on chitosan and apatite. *Crystal Res. Technol.*, (2010), 45, 685–691.

651. Popescu L.M., Rusti C.F., Piticescu R.M., Buruiana T., Valero T., Kintzios S., Synthesis and characterization of acid polyurethane–hydroxyapatite composites for biomedical applications. *J. Compos. Mater.*, (2013), 47, 603–612.

652. Ryabenkova Y., Jadav N., Conte M., Hippler M.F., Reeves-McLaren N., Coates P.D., Twigg P., Paradkar A., Mechanism of hydrogenbonded complex formation between ibuprofen and nanocrystalline hydroxyapatite. *Langmuir*, (2017), 33, 2965–2976.

653. Boanini E., Gazzano M., Rubini K., Bigi A., Composite nanocrystals provide new insight on alendronate interaction with hydroxyapatite structure. *Adv. Mater.*, (2007), 19, 2499–2502.

654. Nastasović, A.B., Ignjatović, N.L., Uskoković, D.P., Marković, D.D., Ekmeščić, B.M., Maksin D.D., Onjia A.E., Determination of thermodynamic interactions of poly(L-lactide) and biphasic calcium phosphate/poly(L-lactide) composite by inverse gas chromatography at infinite dilution. *J. Mater. Sci.*, (2014), 49, 5076–5086.

655. Tsuchiya K., Yoshioka T., Ikoma T., Tanaka J., Chemical interaction between hydroxyapatite and organic molecules in biomaterials. *Ceram. Trans.*, (2010), 210, 531–535.

656. Grossman R.F. Coupling agents. In: *Polymer Modifiers and Additives*, Lutz J.T., Jr., Grossman R.F. (eds), CRC Press: Boca Raton, FL, 2000, pp. 95–106.

657. Chang M.C., Ikoma T., Kikuchi M., Tanaka J., Preparation of a porous hydroxyapatite/collagen nanocomposite using glutataldehyde as a crosslinkage agent. *J. Mater. Sci. Lett.*, (2001), 20, 1199–1201.

658. Sousa R.A., Reis R.L., Cunha A.M., Bevis M.J., Coupling of HDPE/hydroxyapatite composites by silane-based methodologies. *J. Mater. Sci. Mater. Med.*, (2003), 14, 475–487.

659. Dupraz A.M.P., de Wijn J.R., van der Meer S.A.T., Goedemoed J.H., Biocompatibility screening of silane-treated hydroxyapatite powders for use as filler in resorbable composites. *J. Mater. Sci. Mater. Med.*, (1996), 7, 731–738.

660. Dupraz A.M.P., de Wijn J.R., van der Meer S.A.T., de Groot K., Characterization of silane-treated hydroxyapatite powders reinforced for use as filler in biodegradable composites. *J. Biomed. Mater. Res.*, (1996), 30, 231–238.

661. Liao J.G., Wang X.J., Zuo Y., Zhang L., Wen J.Q., Li Y., Surface modification of nano-hydroxyapatite with silane agent. *J. Inorg. Mater.*, (2008), 23, 145–149.

662. Rakmae S., Ruksakulpiwat Y., Sutapun W., Suppakarn N., Effect of silane coupling agent treated bovine bone based carbonated hydroxyapatite on *in vitro* degradation behavior and bioactivity of PLA composites. *Mater. Sci. Eng. C*, (2012), 32, 1428–1436.

663. Marcomini A.L., Rego B.T., Bretas R.E.S., Improvement of the short- and long-term mechanical properties of injection-molded poly(etheretherketone) and hydroxyapatite nanocomposites. *J. Appl. Polym. Sci.*, (2017), 134, 44476.

664. Misra D.N., Adsorption of zirconyl salts and their acids on hydroxyapatite: use of salts as coupling agents to dental polymer composites. *J. Dent. Res.*, (1985), 12, 1405–1408.

665. Carmen A., Rosestela P., Arquimedes K., Gema G., Nohemy D., Yanixia S., Luís, B.J., Characterization of HDPE/HA composites treated with titanate and zirconate coupling agents. *Macromol. Symp.*, (2007), 247, 190–198.

666. Chow W.S., Tham W.L., Ishak Z.A.M., Improvement of microstructure and properties of poly(methyl methacrylate)/hydroxyapatite composites treated with zirconate coupling agent. *J. Thermoplast. Compos. Mater.*, (2012), 25, 165–180.

667. Tham W.L., Chow W.S., Ishak Z.A.M., Effects of titanate coupling agent on the mechanical, thermal, and morphological properties of poly(methyl methacrylate)/hydroxyapatite denture base composites. *J. Compos. Mater.*, (2011), 45, 2335–2345.

668. Shen D., Fang L., Chen X., Tang Y., Structure and properties of polyacrylic acid modified hydroxyapatite/liquid crystal polymer composite. *J. Reinfor. Plast. Comp.*, (2011), 30, 1155–1163.

669. Liu Q., de Wijn J.R., van Blitterswijk C.A., A study on the grafting reaction of isocyanates with hydroxyapatite particles. *J. Biomed. Mater. Res.*, (1998), 40, 358–364.

670. Tanaka H., Yasukawa A., Kandori K., Ishikawa T., Surface modification of calcium hydroxyapatite with hexyl and decyl phosphates. *Colloid Surface A*, (1997), 125, 53–62.

671. Tanaka H., Watanabe T., Chikazawa M., Kandori K., Ishikawa T. T.P.D., FTIR, and molecular adsorption studies of calcium hydroxyapatite surface modified with hexanoic and decanoic acids. *J. Colloid Interf. Sci.*, (1999), 214, 31–37.

672. Borum-Nicholas L., Wilson O.C., Jr., Surface modification of hydroxyapatite. Part I. Dodecyl alcohol. *Biomaterials*, (2003), 24, 3671–3679.

673. Borum L., Wilson O.C., Jr., Surface modification of hydroxyapatite. Part II. Silica. *Biomaterials*, (2003), 24, 3681–3688.

674. Li Y., Weng W., Surface modification of hydroxyapatite by stearic acid: characterization and *in vitro* behaviors. *J. Mater. Sci. Mater. Med.*, (2008), 19, 19–25.

675. Lee S.C., Choi H.W., Lee H.J., Kim K.J., Chang J.H., Kim S.Y., Choi J., Oh K.S., Jeong Y.K., *In-situ* synthesis of reactive hydroxyapatite nanocrystals for a novel approach of surface grafting polymerization. *J. Mater. Chem.*, (2007), 17, 174–180.

676. Sánchez-Salcedo S., Colilla M., Izquierdo-Barba I., Vallet-Regi M., Design and preparation of biocompatible *zwitterionic* hydroxyapatite. *J. Mater. Chem. B*, (2013), 1, 1595–1606.

677. Morita S., Furuya K., Ishihara K., Nakabayashi N., Performance of adhesive bone cement containing hydroxyapatite particles. *Biomaterials*, (1998), 19, 1601–1606.

678. Shinzato S., Nakamura T., Tamura J., Kokubo T., Kitamura Y., Bioactive bone cement: effects of phosphoric ester monomer on mechanical properties and osteoconductivity. *J. Biomed. Mater. Res.*, (2001), 56, 571–577.

679. Dorozhkin S.V., Is there a chemical interaction between calcium phosphates and hydroxypropylmethylcellulose (HPMC) in organic/inorganic composites? *J. Biomed. Mater. Res.*, (2001), 54, 247–255.

680. Kasuga T., Yoshida M., Ikushima A.J., Tuchiya M., Kusakari H., Bioactivity of zirconia-toughened glass-ceramics. *J. Am. Ceram. Soc.*, (1992), 75, 1884–1888.

681. Ehrenfried L.M., Patel M.H., Cameron R.E., The effect of tri-calcium phosphate (TCP) addition on the degradation of polylactide-co-glycolide (PLGA). *J. Mater. Sci. Mater. Med.*, (2008), 19, 459–466.

682. Ehrenfried L.M., Farrar D., Cameron R.E., Degradation properties of co-continuous calcium-phosphate-polyester composites. *Biomacromolecules*, (2009), 10, 1976–1985.

683. Pan J., Han X., Niu W., Cameron R.E., A model for biodegradation of composite materials made of polyesters and tricalcium phosphates. *Biomaterials*, (2011), 32, 2248–2255.

684. Barrett C.E., Cameron R.E., X-ray microtomographic analysis of α-tricalcium phosphate-poly(lactic-*co*-glycolic) acid nanocomposite degradation. *Polymer*, (2014), 55, 4041–4049.

685. Heidemann W., Jeschkeit S., Ruffieux K., Fischer J.H., Wagner M., Krüger G., Wintermantel E., Gerlach K.L., Degradation of poly(D,L) lactide implants with or without addition of calciumphosphates *in vivo*. *Biomaterials*, (2001), 22, 2371–2381.

686. Adamus A., Jozwiakowska J., Wach R.A., Suarez-Sandoval D., Ruffieux K. Rosiak J.M., *In vitro* degradation of β-tricalcium phosphate reinforced poly(L-lactic acid). *Mater. Sci. Forum*, (2012), 714, 283–290.

687. Ahola N., Veiranto M., Rich J., Efimov A., Hannula M., Seppälä, J., Kellomäki M., Hydrolytic degradation of composites of poly(L-lactide-co-ε-caprolactone) 70/30 and β-tricalcium phosphate. *J. Biomater. Appl.*, (2013), 28, 529–543.

688. Dorozhkin S.V., Inorganic chemistry of the dissolution phenomenon: the dissolution mechanism of calcium apatites at the atomic (ionic) level. *Comments Inorg. Chem.*, (1999), 20, 285–299.

689. Dorozhkin S.V., Dissolution mechanism of calcium apatites in acids: a review of literature. *World J. Methodol.*, (2012), 2, 1–17.

690. Furukawa T., Matsusue Y., Yasunaga T., Shikinami Y., Okuno M., Nakamura T., Biodegradation behavior of ultra-high strength hydroxyapatite/poly(L-lactide) composite rods for internal fixation of bone fractures. *Biomaterials*, (2000), 21, 889–898.

691. Furukawa T., Matsusue Y., Yasunaga T., Nakagawa Y., Okada Y., Shikinami Y., Okuno M., Nakamura T., Histomorphometric study on high-strength hydroxyapatite/poly(L-lactide) composite rods for internal fixation of bone fractures. *J. Biomed. Mater. Res.*, (2000), 50, 410–419.

692. Yasunaga T., Matsusue Y., Furukawa T., Shikinami Y., Okuno M., Nakamura T., Bonding behaviour of ultrahigh strength unsintered hydroxyapatite particles/poly(L-lactide) composites to surface of tibial cortex in rabbits. *J. Biomed. Mater. Res.*, (1999), 47, 412–419.

693. Marques A.P., Reis R.L., Hunt J.A., *In vitro* evaluation of the biocompatibility of novel starch based polymeric and composite material. *Biomaterials*, (2002), 6, 1471–1478.

694. Mendes S.C., Bovell Y.P., Reis R.L., Cunha A.M., de Bruijn J.D., van Blitterswijk C.A., Biocompatibility testing of novel starch-based materials with potential application in orthopaedic surgery. *Biomaterials*, (2001), 22, 2057–2064.

695. Habraken W.J.E.M., Liao H.B., Zhang. Z., Wolke J.G.C., Grijpma D.W., Mikos A.G., Feijen J., Jansen J.A., *In vivo* degradation of calcium phosphate cement incorporated into biodegradable microspheres. *Acta Biomater.*, (2010), 6, 2200–2211.

696. Ngiam M., Liao S., Patil A.J., Cheng Z., Chan C.K., Ramakrishna S., The fabrication of nano-hydroxyapatite on PLGA and PLGA/collagen nanofibrous composite scaffolds and their effects in osteoblastic behavior for bone tissue engineering. *Bone*, (2009), 45, 4–16.

697. Liao S.S., Cui F.Z., *In vitro* and *in vivo* degradation of the mineralized collagen based composite scaffold: nanohydroxyapatite/collagen/poly(L-lactide). *Tissue Eng.*, (2004), 10, 73–80.

698. Hasegawa S., Ishii S., Tamura J., Furukawa T., Neo M., Matsusue Y., Shikinami Y., Okuno M., Nakamura T., A 5–7 year *in vivo* study of high-strength hydroxyapatite/poly(L-lactide) composite rods for the internal fixation of bone fractures. *Biomaterials*, (2006), 27, 1327–1332.